blossoming beauty

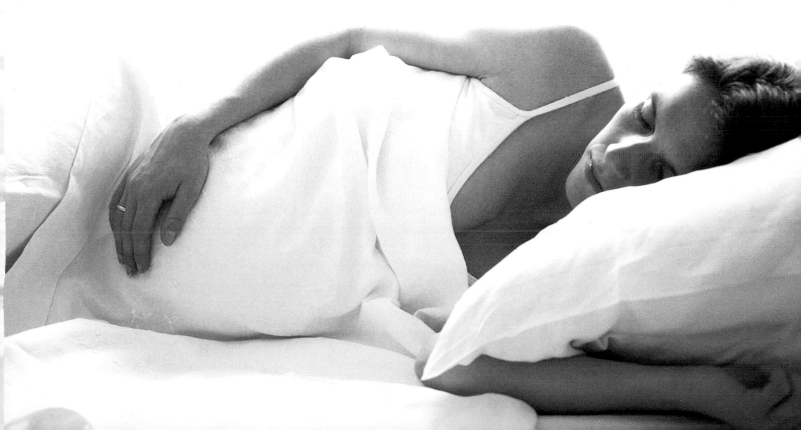

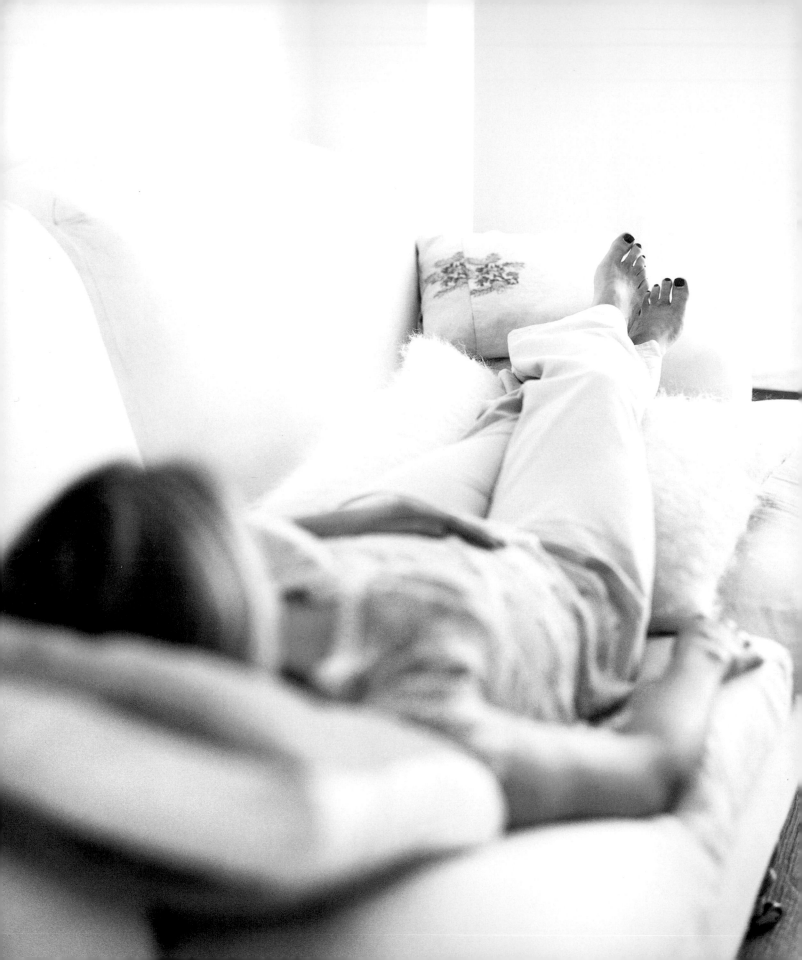

blossoming beauty

wellbeing and looking great during pregnancy

Jo Glanville-Blackburn

with photography by Dan Duchars

RYLAND
PETERS
& SMALL

LONDON NEW YORK

SENIOR DESIGNER Sally Powell
SENIOR EDITOR Henrietta Heald
PICTURE RESEARCH Claire Hector
PRODUCTION Patricia Harrington
ART DIRECTOR Gabriella Le Grazie
PUBLISHING DIRECTOR Alison Starling

ILLUSTRATIONS Javier Joaquin

First published in the USA in 2004 by
Ryland Peters & Small, Inc.
519 Broadway
5th Floor
New York, NY 10012
www.rylandpeters.com

10 9 8 7 6 5 4 3 2 1

Library of Congress Cataloging-in-Publication Data

Glanville-Blackburn, Jo.
 Blossoming beauty : wellbeing and looking great during
pregnancy / Jo Glanville-Blackburn; with photography by
Dan Duchars.
    p. cm.
 ISBN 1-84172-588-9
 1. Pregnancy–Popular works. 2. Prenatal care–Popular
works. 3. Pregnant women–Health and hygiene–Popular
works. 4. Beauty, Personal. I. Title.
 RG525.G5133 2004
 618.2'4–dc22

                                    2003021303

Printed and bound in China.

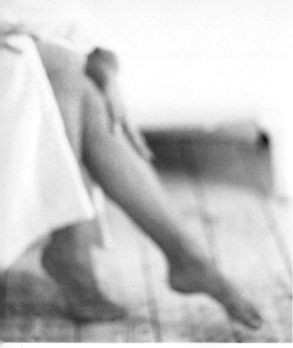

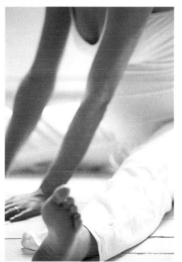

contents

introduction

Ever since the birth of my first child eight years ago, I have wanted to write a book that would help pregnant women to get the most out of pregnancy, from conception to birth and beyond. *Blooming Gorgeous* is the result. It is a book devoted to you, the pregnant woman—a woman who needs to love herself and appreciate herself all the more because a new person will soon be born who will need her as a role model in self-belief.

Pregnancy is the best time to pamper and cosset yourself, to give yourself every bit of attention, because you know that it isn't just for you—your baby will benefit, too. Many pregnancy books dwell on problems and focus on what's happening to the baby, but hey, what about you? It's your body—it's purely on loan—and if you are ever going to get it back in any kind of respectable condition, you need to look after yourself from now on.

My first pregnancy was fantastic. I was the fittest and healthiest I'd ever been. I was incredibly relaxed and so in tune with my body that I have always felt I knew Olivia before she'd even been born. I put it all down to being positive and content. I wanted a baby. It was the right time in my life—I was feeling great in myself and in my relationship. Second time around, it was different. I had a toddler; work was challenging; we were trying to buy a house— there was too much going on. In my third pregnancy, I was more relaxed, but older and far less fit, and I had all sorts of aches and

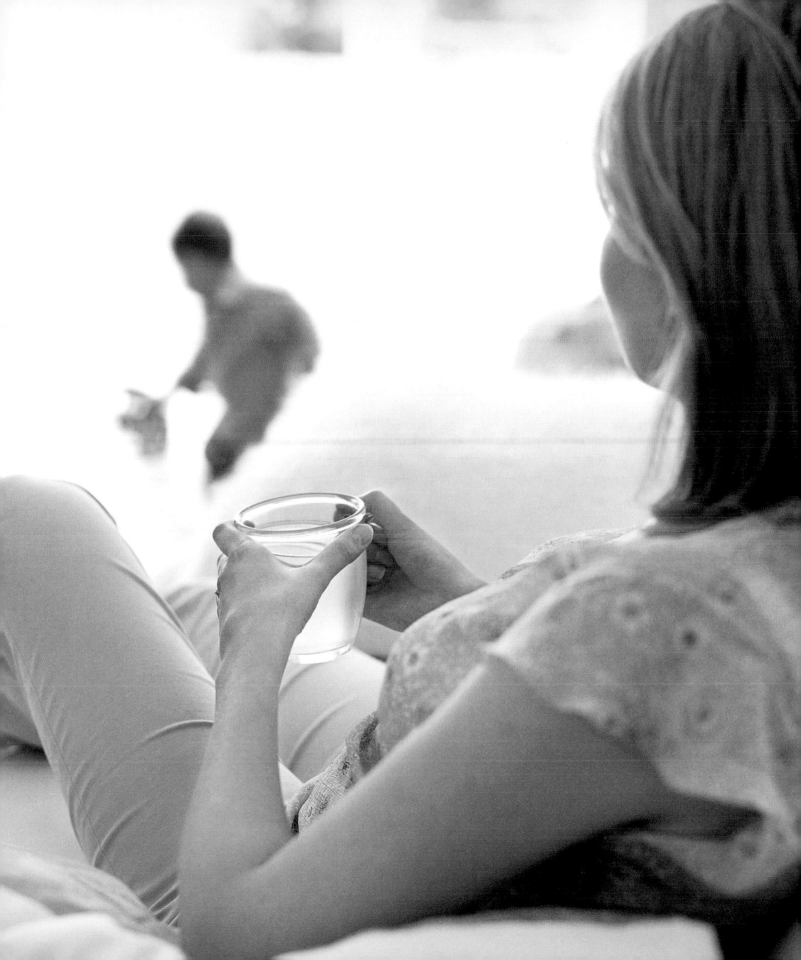

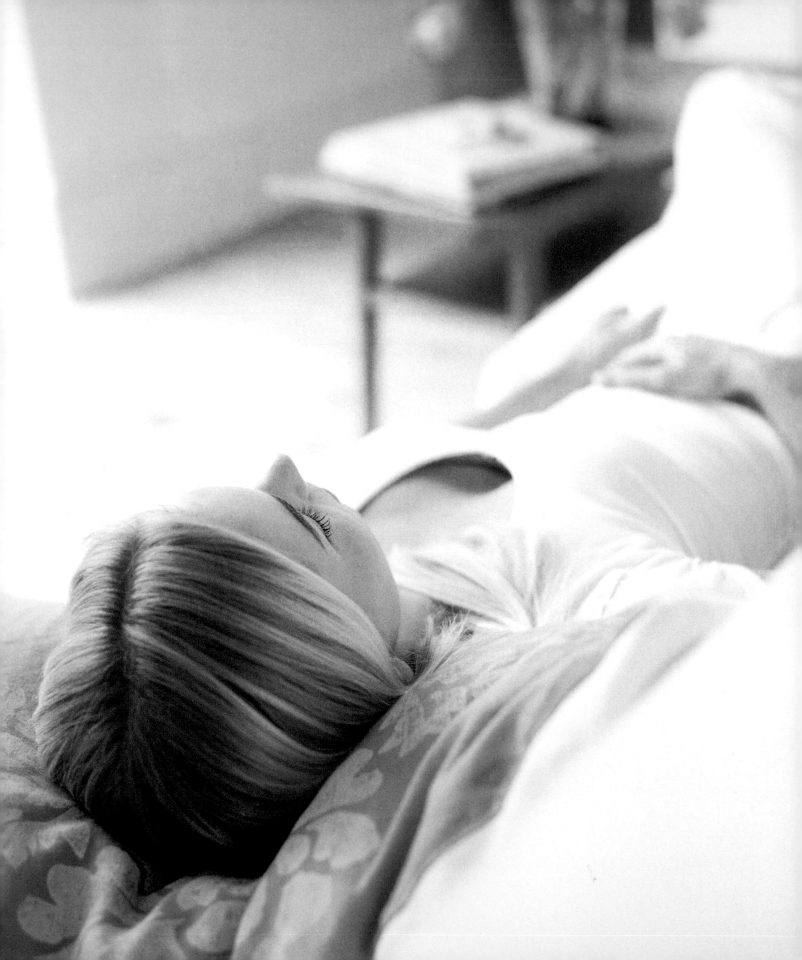

pains. But I was content and had a marvelous birth. And I can honestly say that your positive state of mind is the single most important thing you can give your child for the best start in life. Forget the contest between breastfeeding and bottle-feeding, or between working mom versus at-home mother. If you can stay positive, relaxed, and enthralled by your pregnancy and your children from birth and beyond, you will all benefit.

Pregnancy is an opportunity to treat yourself from top to toe. At a time when you may be feeling apprehensive about the way you are changing physically, a little pampering helps to relax and nurture both body and mind. Think of it as catching a few peaceful moments to yourself, time to help you focus on your baby, and help the baby feel relaxed and nurtured, too. I've included many safe, reliable, trusted, caring treats and remedies for you to try. But, if you are in any doubt, always check with your health practitioner first before trying something new to you in pregnancy.

Each chapter focuses on you, so take what you need from it. What about a foot massage or some visualization techniques? Be inspired to try a little yoga or to make yourself look more radiant, even if you don't feel it yet. Learning the art of relaxation is the key to wellbeing whether you are pregnant or not. A relaxed mother means a relaxed baby—and you can't start soon enough. Don't get stressed about what things you should or shouldn't do while you are pregnant. Have faith in your instincts. Nature is incredibly protective, and trying to live your life in balance is better all around.

preparing for pregnancy

The healthier a woman is at conception, the healthier her
baby will be, so you (and your partner) may need to improve
aspects of your lifestyle before trying to conceive.

A MATTER OF CONCEPTION

Sometimes getting pregnant appears much like the
lottery. Infertility is on the increase, and influenced
by the lifestyle we choose—which may include stress
and poor diet, for example—the odds on conceiving
are getting longer. Given that you are fertile for
only a few days in a month, it is also easy to miss the
opportunity. And, as more and more becomes known
about genetic disorders and birth defects—through
specialized prepregnancy DNA tests or the early CVS
(chorionic villus sampling) chromosome test on the
fetus at 10–12 weeks—the whole business of getting
pregnant may seem harder than you thought.

Whether this is your first or your last baby, or if you
plan several more, it is worth knowing that your health
before conception, and early in pregnancy, matters. If
you are fit and healthy now, it will not only affect the
ease of conception, but is also likely to reduce problems
in pregnancy and keep you feeling and looking good
for the whole nine months and beyond.

LIFESTYLE CHANGES

Not everyone enjoys pregnancy. For some it is a labor
from day one, but this applies more often than not to
women who have started off more stressed, less fit,
and less healthy. However, it's never too late to improve
your state of health. If you haven't yet done so, make
pregnancy a time for a few healthy rituals. In these nine
months your body will naturally try to avoid stimulants
that are not "good," such as coffee, so seize the
moment: if you introduce a few healthy changes to
your lifestyle now, it will benefit you for years to come.

STRATEGIES FOR A HEALTHY PREGNANCY

Look at ways of reducing stress in your life. I've tried
to include as many as possible in this book. Pregnancy
is a great time to learn effective relaxation techniques
that work for you. (We are all individual, so not every
suggestion included in the book will work for you, but
many will.) Learn to say "no" and prioritize things by
importance in your life, and your day.

□ Seek balance in work, rest, and play, for you and
others close to you.

□ Try to take more exercise in the open air, even if it
is no more than brisk walking. If you are fit and have
more strength, suppleness, and stamina from early
pregnancy, the logical consequence is that you will
carry your baby more easily, retain your shape well,
keep going through the labor process, and suffer
less from the niggling aches and pains of pregnancy
such as backache.

□ Start improving your diet simply by choosing
more wholefoods—foods eaten in their natural state
without processing.

□ Take appropriate supplements as recommended by
your doctor. Remember your folic acid; its main role
is to insure that DNA functions properly—otherwise
the fetus may not develop properly. Folic acid helps
to reduce the risk of genetic problems such as spina
bifida, in which the spinal column fails to close properly.
Research in Australia has also found that children born
to mothers who took folic acid supplements during
early pregnancy have a much smaller risk of leukemia.
Women planning pregnancy are generally advised to
take 400 mcg of folic acid a day.

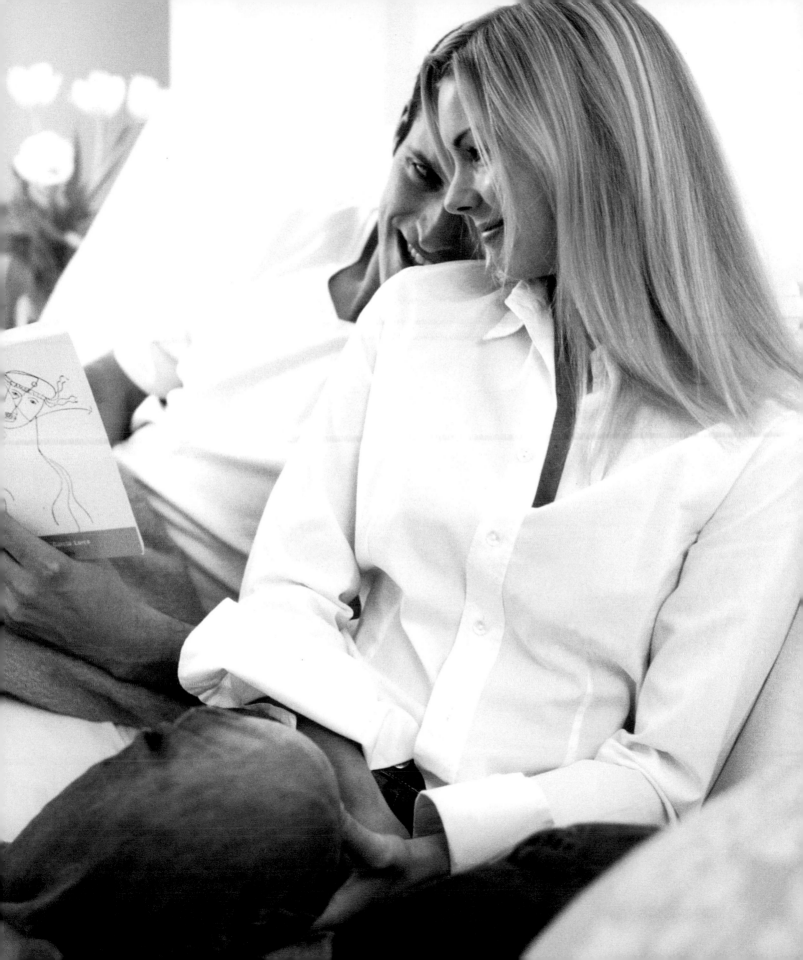

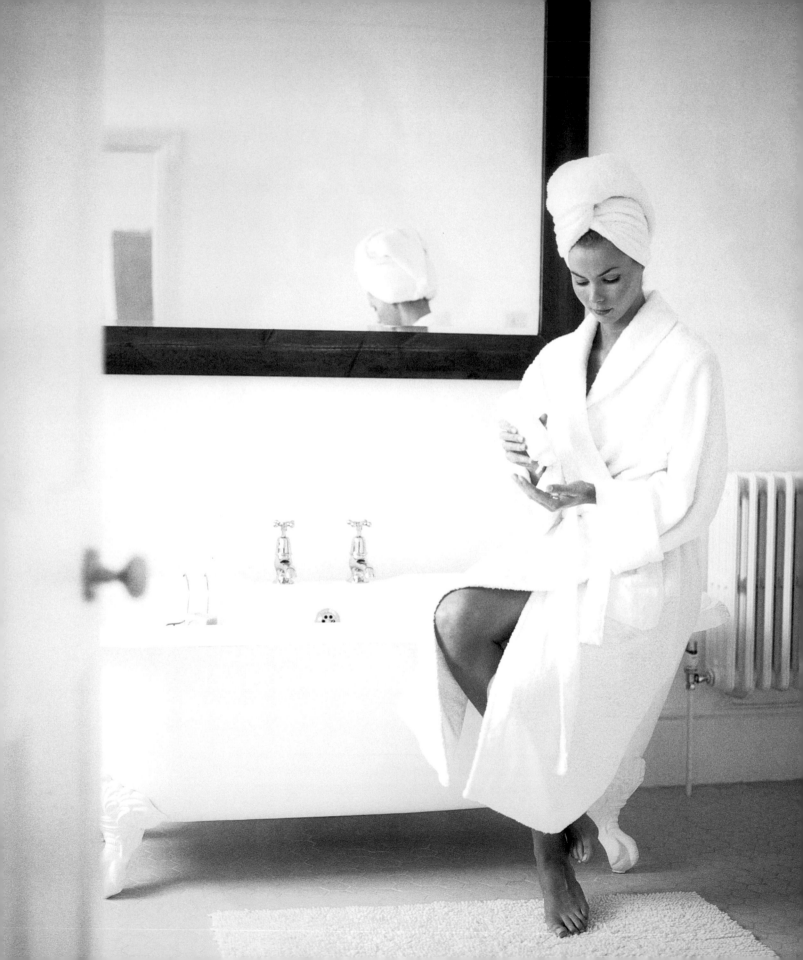

indulge yourself

You are on the threshold of a whole new experience. It won't always be easy, but try to embrace pregnancy for what it is—a time for you to nurture and be nurtured. This interlude will pass swiftly, so make it a series of moments to reflect on with warm memories.

what's changing?

Right now you probably feel not quite your normal self. Although everyone around you may be totally unaware of your pregnancy, you are undergoing some momentous changes, both emotional and physical. You are more sensitive than usual, your buttons keep popping undone— and your jeans won't do up.

MIXED FEELINGS

The demands that a pregnancy makes upon your body can totally sap your energy and make you feel quite exhausted, while turbocharged hormone levels may make you feel overemotional, lacking in focus (which is especially hard if you are working), or even a little depressed.

The mixed feelings associated with early pregnancy can be very unsettling and less of a good start than you might like. So it is reassuring to know that anything you feel—either physically or emotionally—is perfectly normal. While some women sail easily through the early months, most experience a few problems, but these often settle down at around 10 to 14 weeks.

CARING FOR YOUR BREASTS

Your breasts may feel tender and more sensitive from as early as the first 2 to 4 weeks of your pregnancy—even before you have had a pregnancy test. Indeed, tender breasts are often one of the first signs of pregnancy. An aching or tingling sensation in the breasts is extremely common, and very soon your breasts will increase in size due to increased levels of hormones that are preparing your breasts for breastfeeding your baby.

□ Wash your breasts daily, but avoid using soap that is drying to the nipples. Massage a little oil or cream into the skin of your breasts to keep it as supple as possible and help your breasts to regain their shape after the birth. Stretch marks on the breasts are as common during pregnancy as they are in puberty, and while you can't prevent them from happening (you are genetically predisposed to get them—or not), you may help to lessen the effect by nourishing the skin daily so that it retains its elasticity.

□ Breasts contain no muscular tissue, so—if they are to maintain their shape and tone during the next few months and throughout breastfeeding—they will need good support. If you think about all the stretching your skin will be subjected to, you will understand why. The skin around the throat supports the bust, so carry any creams you use over into this area. You should start to adopt a better posture now because rounded shoulders means saggy breasts—and get fitted for a maternity bra early in your pregnancy.

□ Look for sports bras, which may be more flattering than ordinary bras and offer good support; they are also made without an underwire, which can dig into your diaphragm and make you breathless. If your breasts feel heavy, wear a lightweight bra at night for extra comfort. When you take your bra off each night, check your breasts for any marks it may have left during the day. If there are any, you need a bigger cup.

ABDOMINAL CHANGES

At this stage of the pregnancy, your middle probably feels no different from usual. You can't feel the baby moving yet—so apart from the fact that your waist is thickening and your whole midsection (ribcage

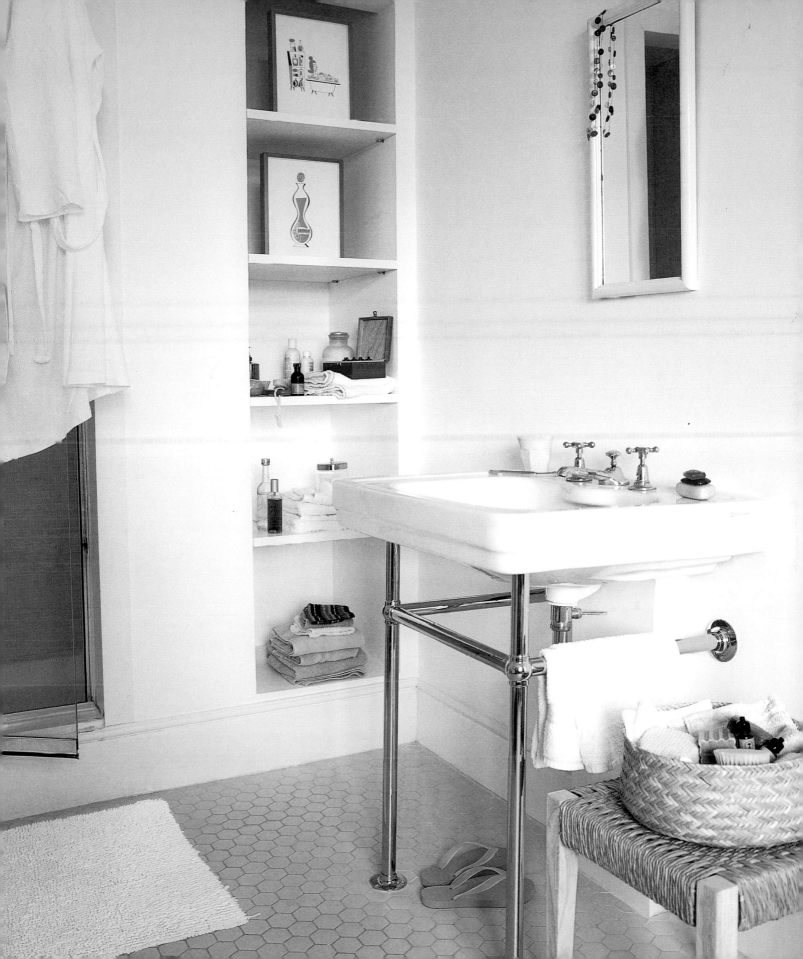

eat what **you feel** like eating—this period doesn't

last long: you have six more months to eat a **healthier** diet

for two based on **quality** rather than quantity

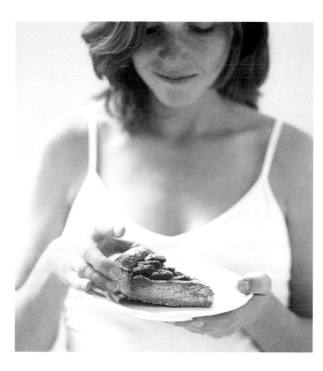

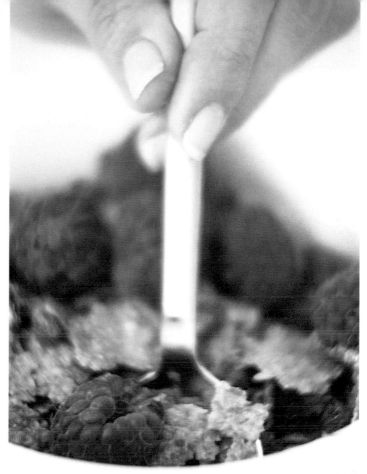

included) is expanding to allow for an extra presence inside—it is easy to forget that you are pregnant.

☐ From the moment you know that you **are** pregnant, massage a skin-nourishing oil into your abdominal area morning and night. Some skincare experts believe that if you don't start this sort of massage until the third or fourth month of pregnancy—by which time the bump starts to show—it is already too late to reduce the likelihood of stretch marks. However, you may be extra-sensitive at this time to the aromas of scented oils and creams, so look at using natural oils on your skin such as vitamin E oil, avocado oil, or sweet almond oil. Many aromatherapy oils should be avoided in the first "delicate" three months of pregnancy.

☐ Even as early as this in the course of a pregnancy, it is worth purchasing comfortable underwear that gives support to your abdomen. Pretty, lacy, all-in-one body suits made from stretch Lycra fabric may feel incredibly comfortable and mold to the shape of your tummy as you expand. If you have heavier breasts, you should wear a supportive bra underneath.

GAINING WEIGHT

Depending on your eating habits, your weight may increase significantly in the early months, especially if you have morning sickness. Strangely, the best cure for morning sickness is to eat—often—and many women worry unduly that the rate at which they gain weight in the first trimester will continue through the pregnancy. But you should succumb to the way you feel—and if eating a certain food such as cake, mash potatoes, or sauerkraut, makes you feel "better," or less nauseous, your body may need that extra bit of carbohydrate or calcium that that food delivers, so right now it is just what you need. Remember to be guided by your body's natural desires. Nature so often knows best.

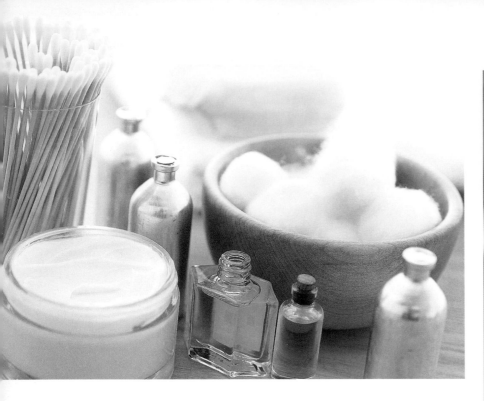

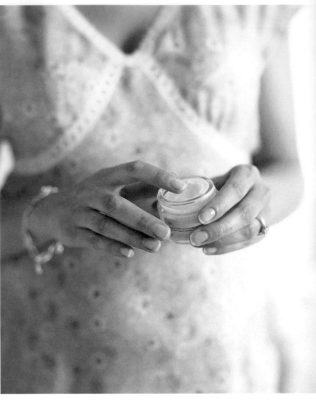

do you look how you feel?

Your skin will probably look its most glowingly healthy while you are pregnant. But not every pregnant woman blooms overnight. For some it takes months—and for a few it never happens at all.

CHANGES TO THE SKIN

Your skin changes in pregnancy in much the same way as it does at other times of hormonal upheaval such as puberty. In pregnancy, the body's level of estrogen—the hormone that gives skin its suppleness, moisture, and smoothness—goes sky high. The result is that, for many of us, by week 14 our skin has improved hugely. Bumps and blemishes disappear, and problems such as acne or oiliness may be greatly reduced. Your skincare regime may become effortless because—no matter what you put on it—your skin can't possibly look better. Or you may find that higher hormone levels make your skin more sensitive than before, and that it becomes either very dry and itchy, or greasy and spotty.

SKIN CARE IN PREGNANCY

Whatever changes you notice, be prepared to adapt your skincare regime for the next few months.

□ If your skin becomes dry, look for creamier cleansers and face masks that you can gently wipe off or remove

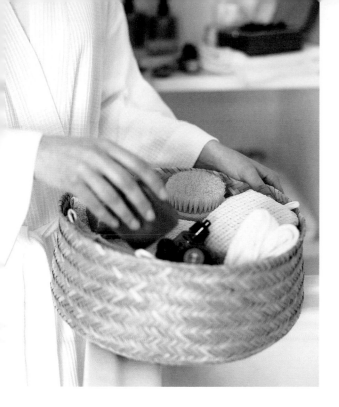

"I have to admit that I loved being pregnant. Just to hear, time and again, those magical words 'Gosh, you look radiant … glowing … vibrant' makes you feel so special. My skin and I had never looked so good."

JO, MOTHER OF OLIVIA, WILLIAM, AND PHOEBE

with a soft cloth, and cream moisturizers that will act as barriers, keeping moisture in the skin and protecting it from the drying effect of the sun.

□ If your skin becomes oily, use oil-based cleansers that dissolve oil and dirt more effectively from the pores, and clay-based masks that help to draw out further impurities. A T-zone control product will minimize shine (many of these contain tiny powder particles that make skin look better immediately). Swap to a light, oil-free moisturizer remember that even oily skin needs moisture. Other beneficial steps include cutting back on stimulants in your diet and doing a little exercise.

□ Your skin may become patchy. Higher levels of the hormones progesterone and estrogen in pregnancy increase the melanin production in skin, creating darker pigmented areas, usually over the face and cheeks. This condition has several names, including melasma, butterfly mask, and the "mask of pregnancy." Mid-toned and olive skins appear to be the most susceptible.

Although the patches eventually fade after the birth, the more your skin has been exposed to the sun, the more stubborn and persistent they tend to be. Wear a high-protection sunscreen to minimize the effect. Subsequent sunbathing may well bring the patches out again, even when you are no longer pregnant, so you will need to protect your skin from ultraviolet exposure.

You can camouflage patchy skin with a concealer, or try using a stick foundation that offers great cover and staying power without making you look too made up. If the pigmentation persists after the birth, and the effect bothers you, ask a qualified dermatologist to give you a mild facial peel that will remove the top surface layers to expose fresher, lighter skin underneath. Seek only qualified professionals to perform this procedure.

□ If you develop bad acne, always consult a doctor before using any medication to treat it in pregnancy. Acne medication may contain ingredients such as vitamin A that could be harmful to your baby.

weeks 1—14   DO YOU LOOK HOW YOU FEEL?

> "You can only be as good as a mother as you are good at mothering yourself."

NOELLA GABRIEL, AROMATHERAPIST AND MOTHER OF KATE

time for you

Motherhood starts not from the day your baby is born but from the moment when you consciously know that you are pregnant. Whether this is your first baby or your fourth, you are now embarking on a nine-month mothering journey. Unless you take good care of yourself, it can be a hard and demanding experience that takes its toll on both mind and body. That is one good reason why you must actively make time to nurture yourself and focus on your wellbeing.

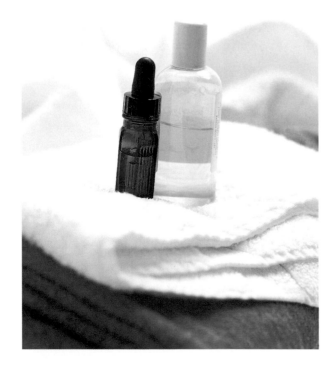

THE IMPORTANCE OF TOUCH

A gentle massage while you are pregnant will not only soothe you but may also help to calm a restless baby. You can enjoy a massage at any time in the pregnancy. Find a sympathetic therapist who will instinctively know which positions are more comfortable. Try any of the following well-established techniques to help you to unwind—and find self-help techniques throughout the book for you to try safely at home.

AROMATHERAPY MASSAGE

Aromatherapy massage (see pages 60–61) uses fragrant essential oils from a wide variety of flowers, plants, and herbs, and its purpose in pregnancy is to help relax your whole being. Key relaxing oils that are considered safe during pregnancy include geranium, neroli, lavender, and sandalwood; jasmine is safe to use after 16 weeks. Pregnant women should avoid all stimulating oils such as clary sage, rosemary, and juniper.

SHIATSU AND ACUPRESSURE

The name shiatsu comes from the Japanese *shi* (meaning finger) and *atsu* (meaning pressure). It is a form of massage using pressure alone on various energy points along meridians associated with the functions of different organs throughout the body.

Acupressure is similar in many ways to shiatsu: this eastern therapy uses the fingers to apply pressure and stimulate specific energy points throughout the body.

REFLEXOLOGY

Reflexology uses massage and finger pressure on the soles of the feet to stimulate specific energy points and help to restore energy flow throughout the body. Seek a professional at all times—applying pressure to specific zones around the ankle may be too stimulating during pregnancy, but very effective before labor.

SWEDISH MASSAGE

Swedish massage, a system of strong, sweeping strokes that helps to boost circulation and lymphatic drainage, is wonderful for relieving tired legs and puffy ankles.

OSTEOPATHY

Osteopathy uses touch and manipulation of the skeletal system to improve your own healing powers and promote inner calm. Women who receive osteopathy during pregnancy may experience less pain in labor.

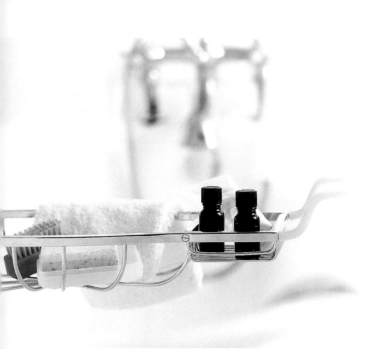

When you are pregnant, you are nurturing a new life that is taking a large amount of energy and substance from you—and you, too, need to feel nurtured. Set yourself a feel-good routine for your pregnancy and practice it daily, morning and evening. It will help you to keep in touch with your body throughout the nine months—and make it easier to cope when trying to get your body back for yourself after the birth.

TEN WAYS TO...*treat yourself*

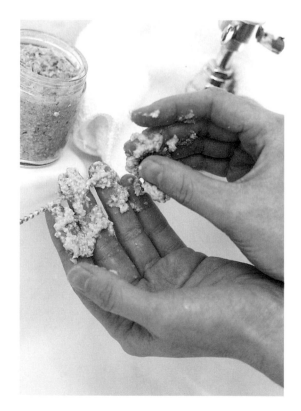

1 Buy an aromatherapy oil diffuser and add a couple of drops of tangerine and grapefruit essential oils to fragrance the air around you and make you feel uplifted and energized first thing in the morning.

2 Lightly exfoliating your skin in the morning is a wonderful way to begin the day, as well as being good for your circulation. Use a grainy body scrub every morning in the shower. Avoiding the abdominal area and breasts entirely, concentrate on your legs and arms. Start from the feet and brush upward. Then start from your hands and brush inward. Remember always to brush toward your heart.

3 Dry body brushing also boosts circulation and minimizes the cellulite that often appears in pregnancy as a result of hormonal upheaval. (It is safe to dry-brush your body in pregnancy.) Brush inward from the feet and hands, avoiding the abdominal area and breasts.

4 Apply a rich body cream to smooth and soothe your skin. You may find that your skin in pregnancy becomes less dry, while other pregnant women find that their skin becomes drier. Set yourself a morning moisturizing routine regardless, so that once you are no longer carrying a baby, your skin will have benefited from the extra care and attention.

5 Start your evening bathing routine by setting the scene. Dim the lights and light a few room candles.

6 Add three drops each of mandarin and rosewood essential oils to still bath water, step in, and immerse yourself in the fragrant warm water.

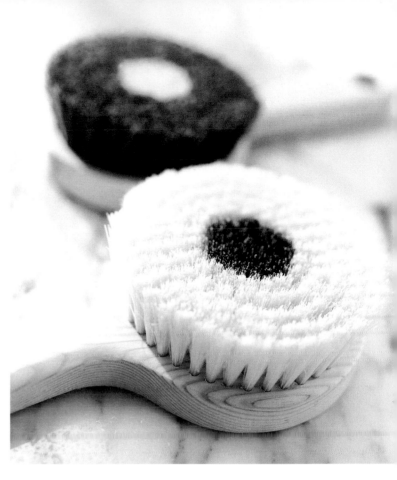

7 Place a soothing eye mask—or a couple of chilled chamomile teabags or slices of cucumber—over your eyes. The ritual of relaxing and pampering every part of your body while you relax is very therapeutic.

8 Take this moment to close your mind down from the pressures and worries of the moment—however big or small—and focus only on yourself and what is happening inside you.

9 Practice this technique inspired by Reiki, a form of "energy healing." Close your eyes and focus your thoughts on a color (silver/white, purple, green, and blue are very positive colors). Breathing calmly, imagine this color entering your body through the top of your head and flooding through into your arms, hands and fingertips, legs and toes. Imagine a warm sensation with the color, and concentrate on keeping this feeling going. Then imagine the color leaving your body; when it leaves the top of your head, open your eyes.

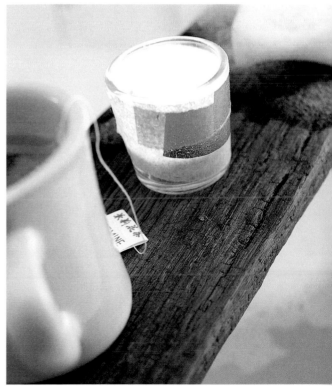

IO When you emerge—ideally feeling rested and calm—pat yourself dry and pamper your skin with plenty of nourishing body oil.

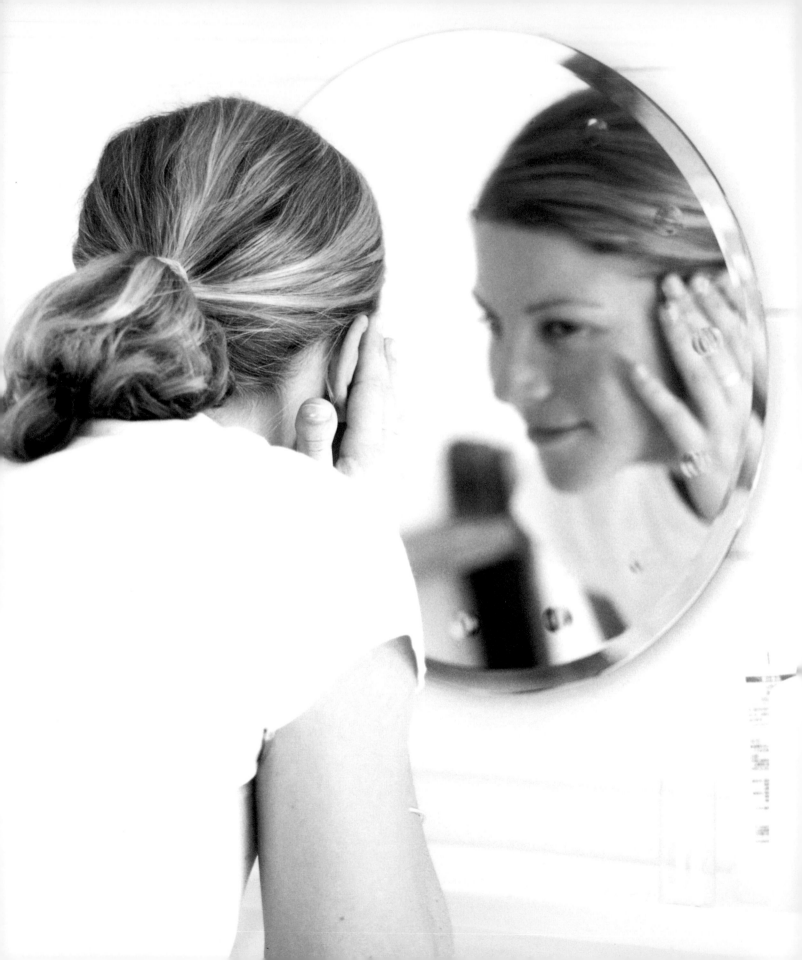

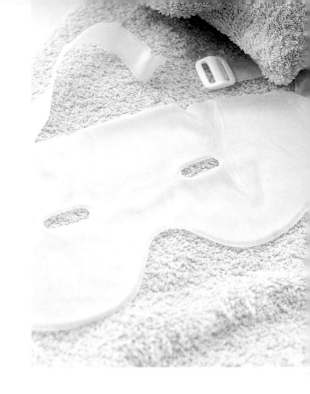

how to hide it

The chances are that during the early weeks of pregnancy you may be trying to conceal your good news—from either the family or the boss, or both. By the end of the first trimester, they will probably have started to notice some changes in you, but in the meantime there are several tactics you can use to keep them guessing.

TELL-TALE SIGNS

The two great "giveaways" in early pregancy are a thickening waistline and exhaustion. There are plenty of ways to disguise these or remedy the consequences.

EXPANDING WAISTLINE

It is easy to cover up a pregnancy in winter under layers of clothing, but in summer, too, you can dress cleverly— certainly until you reach 14 weeks.

□ Opt for bias-cut dresses that don't dig into the waist and hips. Anything tight around your waist will be uncomfortable and may make you feel more nauseous.

□ Buy maternity hosiery as soon as possible—and banish uncomfortable tight waistbands.

□ A mid- to long-length cardigan makes you look longer rather than wider, and can mask a thickening waist.

□ Around your neck and shoulders, wear a long floaty scarf or wrap (patterns and tassels are good, too) that ends below your hips. It will sway as you walk—so those around you should be less inclined to make comments about your changing shape.

□ Choose maternity wear that cleverly disguises itself as fashionable clothing—a leather skirt with stretchy bands around the bump, for example.

SHORT OF SLEEP?

If it's bags under the eyes that are giving you away, try the anytime, anywhere pick-me-up described below.

□ Sit relaxed in a chair, with your elbows on a table in front of you. Lightly interlock your fingers and place both thumbs between your brows. Let your head rest on your thumbs, lightly bearing the pressure. Hold for a count of five, then repeat in six steps along the brow, gradually moving your thumbs apart. Finish by sitting up and gently pressing with your middle fingers along the delicate area beneath each eye.

□ For a quick fix, soak and chill two chamomile teabags (used ones are fine). Lie down and place the teabags on your closed eyelids, leaving them there for 10 minutes.

□ Take time out for a face mask. It is a great way to force yourself to take a rest and lie still for ten minutes.

□ Find a yellow-toned concealer and apply only where you need it to hide darkness under the eyes.

□ Take the heat out of skin to reduce puffiness. Top beauty therapist Janet Filderman suggests wrapping a small ice cube in a handkerchief and gliding it over your cheek from the inside corner of the nose to the ear and down the side of the face to just under the jaw. Repeat on the other side.

"The first time I heard her tiny heartbeat
I knew it was real. It felt incredible to think
something so tiny and strong was growing
inside me since I still barely showed that
I was pregnant from the outside."

GAIL, MOTHER OF DREW AND MARTHA

nature's way

**Your body is amazing. At this moment it is creating the most
harmonious environment for your baby, and Mother Nature—
that is, your body and your newly heightened senses—are
tuned in from the word Go to protect and preserve that tiny
being. It's only natural, after all, and it's good to be aware of
the way your body subconsciously protects from the outside in.**

A BALANCING ACT

Although from time to time it may feel as if you have
been invaded, don't forget that your body is in the
middle of an amazing balancing act. You should feel
back in control by the 14th week—by which time the
baby will be fully developed and simply needing time
to grow. At times of anxiety in your pregnancy, take a
few quiet moments to dwell on the beauty of it all.

MISCARRIAGE

Sadly, the body sometimes rejects the pregnancy for
one reason or another, resulting in miscarriage. It is
estimated that as many as 25 percent of pregnancies
end in miscarriage in the first 20 weeks. If the baby
dies after 20 weeks, it is known as stillbirth. The loss
of a baby early on is no less heartbreaking than at
any other stage in the pregnancy. This is a time to
seek support from those around you.

SMELL AND TASTE

In pregnancy you have a particularly heightened sense
of smell and taste, which are inextricably linked with
each other. Right now you may find that your body is
naturally turning you away from strong aromas (of
certain paints and perfumes, for example) and tastes
(such as the taste of coffee, alcohol, or cigarette
smoke). Let your senses be your guide. Your body is
reacting to the new life that has invaded—and, well,
pretty much taken over.

So remember—whatever you do for your body right
now has to be with you in mind, too—because that
baby is going to look after itself—so long as you look
after yourself.

Your heightened sense of smell can even affect the
perfume you wear, so much so that many women
can't bear to wear their usual scent, opting instead for
more natural aromas—or nothing at all. According

to experts in perfumery, this is nature's clever way of protecting us, making sure we surround ourselves only with positive, natural aromas. If you really miss your perfume—though the chances are you won't—you may well find that you can better tolerate the scented body lotion version instead.

COMMON SYMPTOMS

Common symptoms in early pregnancy that affect you but often don't rate as important because they don't harm the baby are:

□ A bloated, irrational feeling like PMS.

□ Tender breasts, or painful nipples in cold weather.

□ Hot flashes and dizziness—a need for fresh air.

□ A taste for strong flavors—most typically pickles/sauerkraut.

□ Nausea and vomiting or a distaste for certain smells or foods.

□ A need to urinate more frequently, due to your expanding uterus pressing on your bladder.

□ Digestive upsets such as constipation or gas.

□ Excessive saliva or a metallic taste in your mouth.

□ Breakthrough bleeding when your period would have been due.

□ Lifeless hair and greasy skin or spots.

□ Pulling pains at the sides of the abdomen caused by the round ligaments stretching as the uterus moves.

BLEEDING

Up to 30 percent of women experience some kind of bleeding during the first three months of pregnancy, but research shows that, while women who bleed during the first trimester are more likely to have a miscarriage than women who don't, the risk is much lower than had been thought.

According to research from 15 medical institutions in the U.S., the risk of miscarriage after bleeding is put at 5 percent (rising to 20 percent if the bleeding occurs very early in the first trimester). But, if you bleed in the first three months, you are more likely to have

complications such as premature birth and high blood pressure. And the more blood there is, the higher the risk of complications. Consult your health practitioner about any bleeding at any stage in your pregnancy.

BOOKING IN

As you near the end of the first trimester, you will need to make an appointment to book in with your chosen hospital. This will be the longest medical appointment during your pregnancy. Your weight, height, and blood pressure will be measured. A blood sample will be taken to establish your blood type and check for anemia or HIV (the latter is usually an optional test). You will be asked to provide a urine sample to check for the presence of protein or glucose. And you will also be asked about your family health and lifestyle history. Seek advice on anything you are not sure about.

You may also be given a dating scan that precisely predicts your baby's due date, especially if you are not sure when your last period was, or if you are having the CVS chromosome test, which needs to be carried out when you are between 10 and 12 weeks' pregnant.

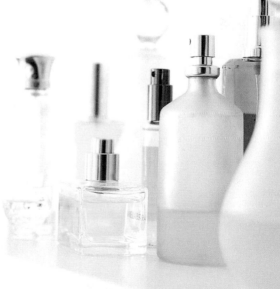

you've probably heard it all before,
but **water** is **important** for **vitality**,
clear **skin**, and bright **eyes**

changing habits

Pregnancy is a good time to start listening to your body and becoming more in tune with it. Things you did before—daily tasks and regular habits, some good, some bad— may all need to change now that you are pregnant. But most of the changes will benefit you as well as your baby.

ALCOHOL

Traditionally, doctors have advised women to avoid alcohol during pregnancy, and since many pregnant women lose the desire to drink anyway, it is often no great hardship to give up.

Heavy drinking during pregnancy can cause fetal alcohol syndrome, a condition that results in birth defects and learning disabilities. Most medical experts now advise pregnant women to avoid drinking alcohol altogether, though an occasional (single-unit) drink is acceptable. Again, trust your instincts. If you have always enjoyed a glass of wine and still desire it, you should decide what to do. Seek help if you find it hard to avoid alcohol in excess during pregnancy.

COFFEE

Pregnant women who drink too much coffee are more likely to have a restless baby, and recent research also suggests that it can do further harm if taken in large quantities. Researchers from Aarhus University Hospital in Denmark surveyed more than 18,000 pregnant women and found that the risk of stillbirth increased with the amount of coffee drunk during pregnancy. Women who drank four to seven cups a day had an 80 percent increased risk of stillbirth, compared with women who drank no coffee at all. Those who drank eight or more cups a day had a 300 percent greater risk. Most pregnant women find that they are automatically turned off coffee (good old Mother Nature stepping in again)—but, if you are not, it is strongly recommended that you cut back on the amount you drink, if not avoid it completely.

SMOKING

Smoking is not only detrimental to your health and fitness; it can also affect your baby before, during, and after pregnancy.

Smokers have a higher incidence of miscarriage and an increased likelihood of bleeding in pregnancy. The poor oxygen levels delivered to the fetus may mean that babies of smokers are born smaller, less developed, and more prone to breathing problems such as asthma than those of nonsmokers. Smokers are also more likely to drink alcohol during pregnancy. Try to use your pregnancy as a real reason to give up. Seek advice if you cannot manage to quit on your own.

WATER

Drink more water. You may have heard it all before, but water is important for vitality, clear skin, and bright eyes, and helps offset the fluid retention that you may suffer from over the next few months. Don't wait until you are thirsty—aim to drink at least six 8-ounce glasses (1.5 litres) of water daily. It is vital to drink more while you are breastfeeding, too. Drink uncarbonated water whenever possible; try commercially flavored versions for variety.

eating for two

It's funny how food takes on a whole new level of importance when you are expecting a baby. Many women become more aware in pregnancy of what they are eating, but especially during the early months, it is all too easy to fall into the comfort-eating mentality simply because food is often a good remedy for nausea.

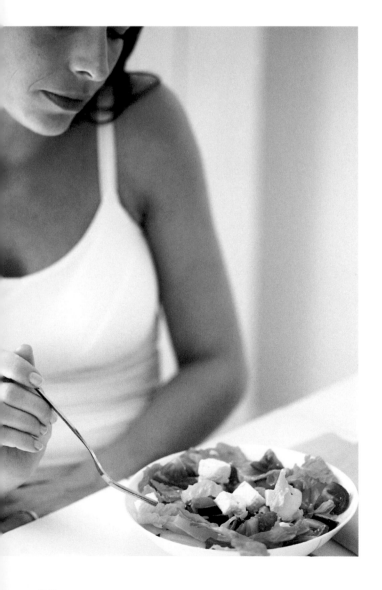

AIMING FOR QUALITY

When pregnant, you are providing nutrition for yourself and for your developing baby. Don't go overboard on quantity, but aim for quality: a varied, high-protein diet rich in the vitamins and minerals that will benefit your own body as much as your baby's. Eat fresh wholefoods whenever you can. In winter, when salads may be less appetizing, don't forget to eat plenty of vegetables, lightly steamed or lightly broiled with olive oil.

WHAT DO I NEED?

Don't resist—your body knows what it needs—but try to eat what you eat in moderation, bearing in mind the following constituents of a healthy diet in pregnancy.
☐ At least 70g protein a day from meat, fish, poultry, cooked eggs, or nuts and legumes. This is particularly important if you feel weak and tired much of the time.
☐ Complex carbohydrates such as wholewheat bread and whole grains. Avoid simple carbohydrates such as sugar, white flour, and refined rice.
☐ Foods with a high fiber content such as legumes, nuts, wholewheat bread, vegetables, and fruit.
☐ The right fats, such as fish oils, olive oil, and flaxseed oil. Avoid the transfats found in many soft margarines, low-fat spreads, and spreadable butter.
☐ Dairy products such as milk and cheese, whose calcium is essential for the baby's bone development.

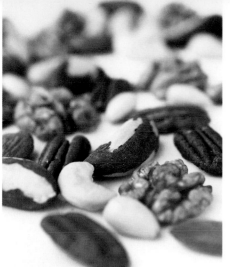
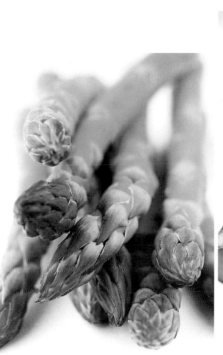
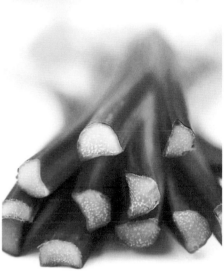

OILY FISH

Increase your intake of oily fish such as salmon, tuna, mackerel, and sardine. They contain a fat called docosohexaenoic acid (DHA), which is vital in the development of the brain in pregnancy and the first weeks of life. A Norwegian study gave a group of women DHA-rich cod liver oil (10 ml/2 tsp per day) from the 18th week of pregnancy until their babies were age three months. Four years later, the children's intelligence was assessed, and the children born to mothers who had taken cod liver oil supplements were found to solve problems and process information better than another group whose mothers had taken corn oil supplements (containing no DHA). An earlier study showed that children of women who took cod liver oil in pregnancy are 70 percent less likely to develop diabetes.

IRON

Aim to take about 30 mg of iron a day to prevent anemia. Iron is found in dried apricots, raisins, dates, prunes, spinach, poultry, beef, and molasses.

VITAMIN C

Increasing your intake of vitamin C by eating fruit such as kiwis and oranges may help to reduce the risk of premature birth. Scientists at the University of North Carolina found that the lower the intake of vitamin C before and during pregnancy, the greater the risk of waters breaking prematurely. The researchers argue that vitamin C is important for the production of collagen, which gives the fetal sac its strength. Research has also shown that women with very low levels of vitamin C are nearly four times as likely to suffer from pre-eclampsia.

DIETARY SUPPLEMENTS

You should continue to take folic acid supplements (see page 10) throughout early pregnancy as advised by your doctor. Many doctors also recommend a daily multivitamin and multimineral supplement that has been specially designed for pregnant women. Such a supplement is particularly appropriate if any of the following applies to you:

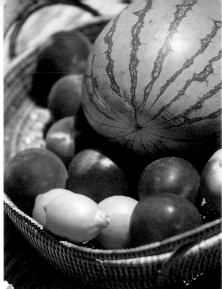

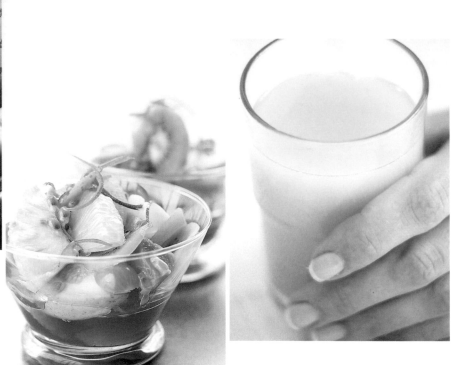

□ You are allergic to certain foods such as wheat or cows' milk.

□ You are on a strict diet for health reasons (because you have developed gestational diabetes, for example).

□ You are an adolescent mother-to-be, and as such are still growing along with your baby.

□ You have previously lost a baby through miscarriage or stillbirth.

□ You are pregnant with more than one baby.

□ You are working hard or are under a lot of stress.

□ You continue to smoke or drink alcohol in pregnancy.

WHAT DON'T I NEED?

Pregnancy is a time to cut back on sugary carbohydrates that can add pounds to your weight while offering no nutritional benefit to you or your baby.

□ Beware of the sugar trap after the birth, when you may be breastfeeding or feeling tired and seemingly in need of the quick energy fix provided by simple carbohydrates. Sugar will not only cause weight gain,

even if you are breastfeeding, but may also exacerbate any mood swings you may have after the birth.

□ Avoid paté, soft cheese, undercooked meat, raw eggs, and refrigerated smoked seafood, any of which may harbor harmful bacteria. Paté and soft cheeses (including goat and sheep cheese) may contain the listeria bacterium, which increases the risk of miscarriage and stillbirth. Meat and eggs should always be cooked thoroughly and served hot. You can also help avoid contamination by always washing hands, knives, and cutting board after handling uncooked foods, and by always washing raw vegetables.

LOSING WEIGHT

Some pregnant women may find that they lose weight during the first trimester. Do not worry about the baby; it will take everything it needs nutritionally from you. However, if you suffer from morning sickness (see pages 34–35), make sure you start to build yourself up once the sickness has passed.

eating a nutritious diet is **energizing** and **nourishes** your whole **body** from within—create **delicious** fruit drinks, tasty **salads**, and healthy **snacks**

morning sickness

Morning sickness is the common term used to describe any type of nausea or vomiting experienced in these first weeks of pregnancy, often in weeks 8 to 12.

THE SIGN OF A HEALTHY PREGNANCY?

Up to 70 percent of pregnant women suffer from morning sickness, varying from queasiness first thing in the morning to a nausea that comes and goes during the day to a full-on head-down-the-pan for temporary relief. Morning sickness has historically been held to signify a healthy pregnancy—"a sign that your pregnancy hormones are doing their job"—but there are still a third of pregnant women who never experience it and have a perfectly healthy baby.

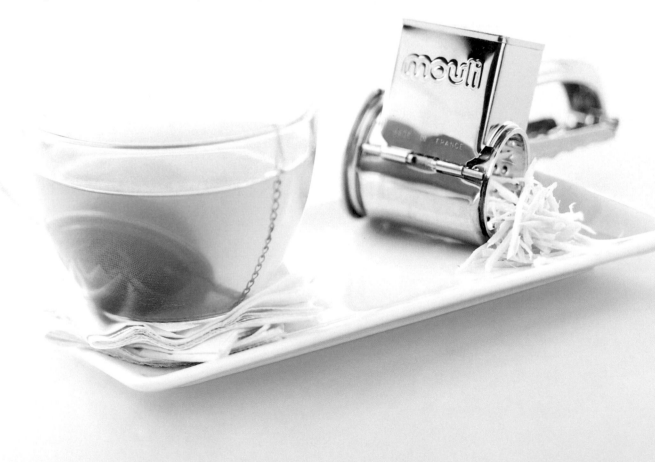

REMEDIES FOR MORNING SICKNESS

Morning sickness can have any one of a number of causes, including hormonal changes, low blood sugar, low blood pressure, or a diet low in vitamin B6 and iron.

□ Eat little and often. You usually feel worse if your stomach is empty, so the trick is to top yourself up with nutritional snacks that curb that empty feeling.

□ Keep a pack of plain crackers by your bed and nibble on a couple before you get up in the morning. This may help prevent the onset of sickness or lessen its effect.

□ Drink plenty of fluids, but take them slowly.

□ Peppermint and ginger are both known to help relax the digestive system. Make a tea of either one and sip slowly at regular intervals without food.

□ Try gingersnaps, or anything with real ginger in it (grated fresh ginger in a glass of hot water).

□ Avoid strong aromas and perfumes.

□ Certain foods and drinks such as salmon, peppers, coffee, or spicy foods can trigger nausea. Either their taste or their smell can trigger sickness. Avoid cooking food with strong aromas.

□ If your sickness is due to tiredness, it may be worse in the early evening. Try to get a rest in the middle of the day. Use the first-aid room at your place of work, or go and sit on a park bench at lunchtime with your feet up.

□ Applying pressure to the Pericardium 6 meridian on the wrist is a recognized treatment for both morning sickness and travel sickness. With palm facing upward, place three fingers from the other hand next to each other across your wrist, with your ring finger resting on the wrist crease. Press where the index finger rests for 5–10 seconds. You could wear travel "seasickness" bands around your wrists, but these may feel too tight

□ The homeopathic remedy Sepia 30C may help the kind of sickness experienced in the afternoon, which is worse with certain smells and makes you irritable.

□ For severe nausea, try Nux vomica 30C, or Ipecacuana 30C three times a day for five days.

□ Slippery elm herbal tablets or powder may help to soothe your stomach.

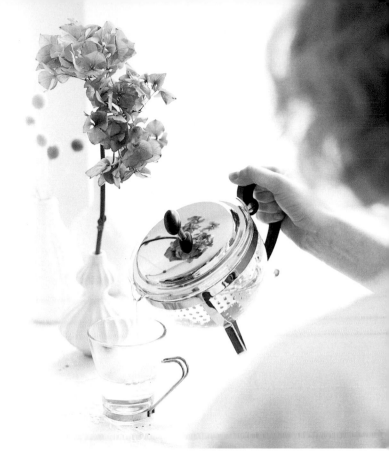

"My husband did all the cooking for me at the beginning—chopping certain vegetables made me feel sick. At times it was so bad that I couldn't even stand to be in the same room."

MARY, MOTHER OF JEMIMA AND ELEANOR

□ The thunderbolt pose in yoga relaxes the intestinal muscles. Kneel upright on the floor, feet behind, knees together, heels apart but big toes crossed. Lower your bottom to your feet, sitting between the heels. Place your hands palm down on your forelegs and relax the tummy muscles, breathing rhythmically. Repeat, and practice after meals to prevent indigestion, too.

□ Eat more foods rich in iron such as wholegrains, figs, prunes, and broccoli, and take a vitamin B6 supplement.

posture in pregnancy

It's that classic posture that many an expectant mother adopts: shoulders back, hands on hips, elbows out, tummy out. No doubt about it ... you're pregnant. But poor posture and tension while carrying an extra load place undue strain on your back in pregnancy.

KEEPING A STRAIGHT BACK

High levels of progesterone in pregnancy cause the ligaments to soften and stretch to make room for the growing baby. This affects the spinal ligaments, putting strain on the back and hips. Also, as the baby's weight increases, the mother's center of gravity moves forward over the legs, making her arch her back to compensate. This puts added strain on the back muscles and results in an aching back. The solution is to avoid slouching. Whether you are walking, standing, or sitting, keep your back in a straight line as often as is comfortable.

Try this Pilates stretching technique to help you to adopt a straighter back. Stand against a wall with your entire back pressed against it. Then slowly roll your neck and upper back downward, as if you are lifting each vertebra off the wall as you roll down—then roll back up again. Only go as far as is comfortable.

OTHER TIPS FOR GOOD POSTURE

□ Don't bend or stoop to reach the ground; sit or kneel instead to bring your whole body down to floor level. If you already have one or more children, it is important not to overstretch yourself by stooping to lift them. Before attempting to pick up one of your children, sit yourself down to the child's level .

□ When lifting things, squat down and hold the object as close to your body as possible. When you stand up again, keep your back straight and use your leg muscles to do the lifting. Don't try to lift anything heavy.

□ Avoid standing with all your weight on one leg; try to keep your weight evenly distributed.

□ Avoid wearing high-heeled shoes. They may be the height of fashion, but you can afford to wait a few more months. There are lots of pretty inch-high styles that are much better for you.

□ Sleep on a soft mattress, on a firm base (not sprung). This is the best type of bed for anyone with back problems, pregnant or not. From six or seven months, you may want to relieve the pressure on your spine while you sleep by lying on your side with one pillow between your legs and another supporting your back.

□ When getting up from lying on the floor, roll onto your knees and use your thigh muscles rather than your abdominal muscles to lift you up.

throughout pregnancy you will need an **abundance of pillows** and cushions to keep you comfortable

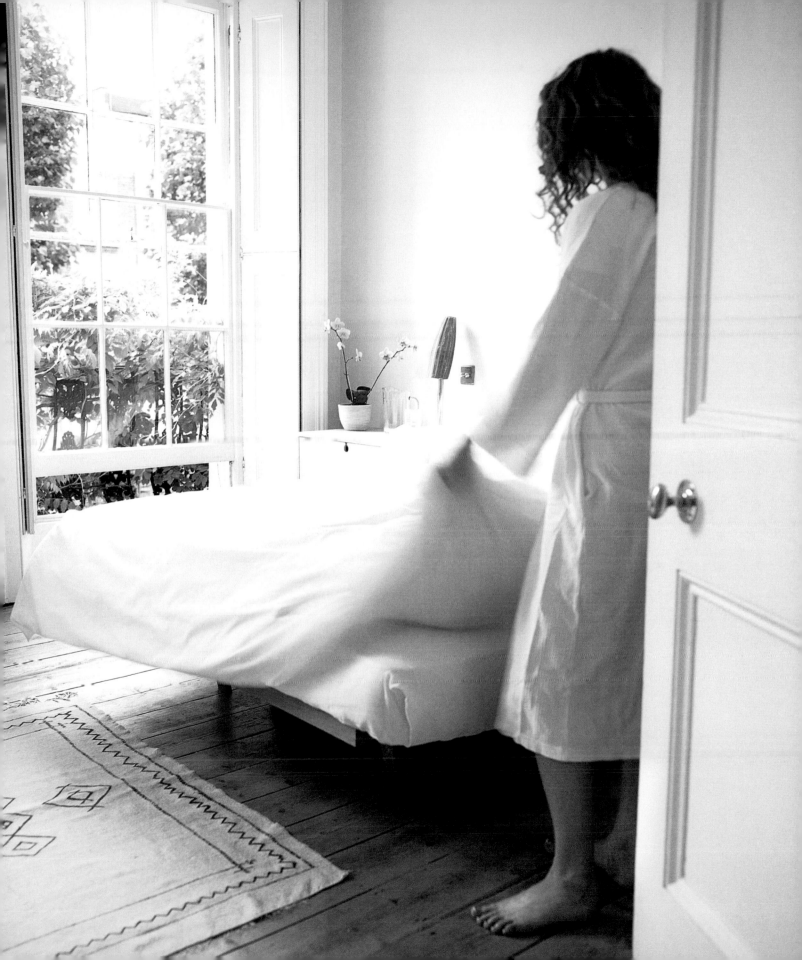

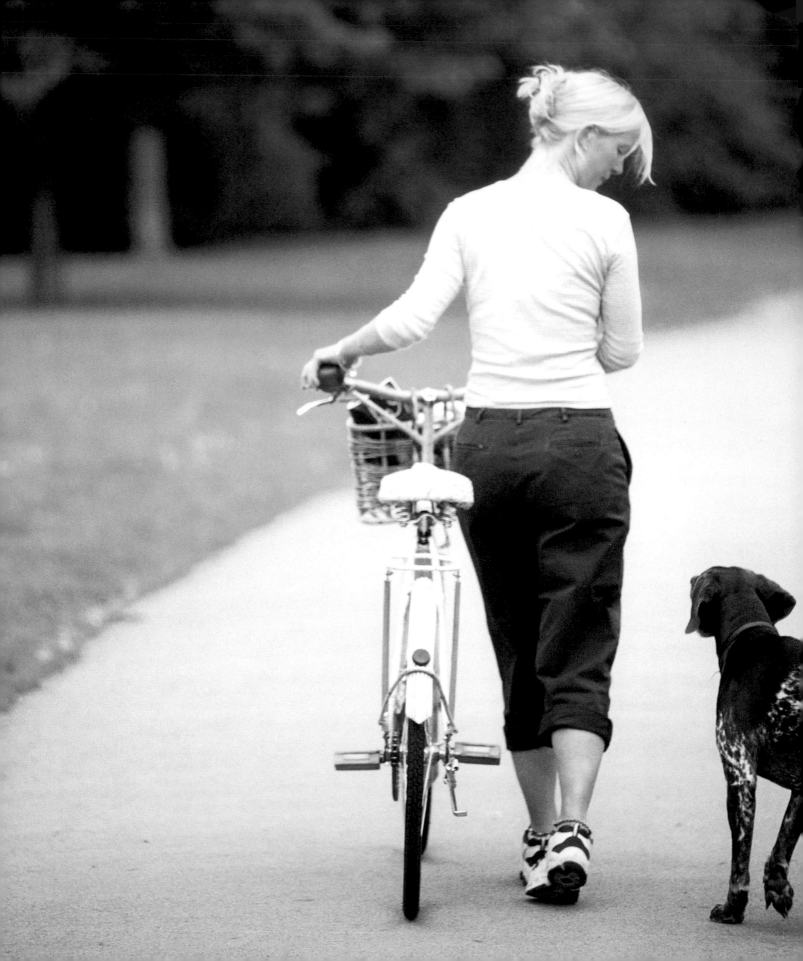

"I kept doing the same sports I'd done before I was pregnant and felt fabulous throughout. I had a very quick birth."

LARA, MOTHER OF ALEXANDER AND EVIE

exercise in pregnancy

Believe it or not, exercise during pregnancy will calm and revitalize both your mind and body. Better still, experts now agree that you'll have a healthier, happier, fitter baby. Just remember to take it easy.

OVERCOMING FEARS

Previously fit from working out three times a week, I was instantly scared of exercising when I became pregnant with my first daughter, Olivia. What if the precious "bean" got squashed as I did another ab crunch? And, if I felt breathless, how would the baby be feeling? Suddenly, experiencing a bit of pain for not much gain worried me senseless, and I abruptly stopped exercising. After a couple of months of slothfulness, I discovered walking ... and I walked and walked.

With baby number two, there was more to do. Excess weight left behind from the extremely large amounts of carbohydrate I consumed while breastfeeding (yes, I've been there) piled on the pounds. But I discovered yoga and Pilates, and rediscovered swimming.

WHY IT'S GOOD TO EXERCISE

Pregnancy, labor, and the initial months after birth can place huge demands on your body, so try to stay active. Regular exercise increases energy levels, so the more you can prepare yourself physically, the better you will feel. "Mild exercise in pregnancy encourages good blood flow," says leading personal trainer Matt Roberts,

"which means better circulation and less likelihood of getting swollen feet and legs, or varicose veins." It also strengthens your muscles (remember your abdominal muscles support your back and will prevent back pain), promotes a strong pelvic floor, eases tension, and helps prevent future problems. And, it will help you to regain your shape more quickly after the birth.

You should feel comfortable and happy about any exercise you undertake in pregnancy. Get advice and be supervised by a fitness professional when possible, and don't try to do an exercise that you did not do before you were pregnant. If your muscles were not strong enough before pregnancy, they are less likely to cope with the extra strain—and you could end up injuring your back and your abdominal muscles.

WHAT CAN I DO?

As a general rule, it is fine to continue with exercise you did before you became pregnant—just take everything a bit more slowly (and see also what to avoid, page 40). But this is not the time to start trying out an exercise that is wholly new to you, with the exception of swimming. "Swimming is perfect," says Matt Roberts.

and movement in pregnancy
is invigorating to mind and body; no matter what
you choose to do, do something **outdoors**

"It's a great all-round aerobic exercise that you can do at your own pace, and because you are buoyant in the water, it exerts no load-bearing strain on the body."

Bicycling, walking, and floor exercises such as squats or lunges help to keep the body flexible and mobile. Yoga-based exercises (see pages 70–73) are designed to improve suppleness and flexibility, and they also encourage deep breathing—which is useful practice for labor. Always listen to your body. If anything at any time doesn't feel right, STOP.

WHAT CAN'T I DO?

The bottom line is: avoid overdoing it. Keep active, but never exercise to the point where you run out of breath or can't speak while moving. Always tell a fitness instructor that you are pregnant, and seek advice if you are unsure about anything. Here's what to avoid:

□ Running or jogging puts too much strain on the pelvic floor and around the uterus, especially during the third trimester when there is already an incredible amount of strain and pressure on this area.

□ Any exercise that involves lying flat on your back with feet raised—this position can cut off the blood supply to the fetus. (Always raise your head with a cushion or pillow.)

□ Leg curls and extensions—again, these raise blood pressure too quickly.

□ Horse riding, skiing, and waterskiing—to name a few of the sports where you run the risk of falling badly and injuring your abdominal area.

□ Any vigorous exercise that raises both your blood pressure and body temperature excessively; this can be overwhelming to a fetus.

□ "Avoid too much stretching," warns Matt. "Pregnancy releases relaxing hormones which tend to soften joints; so if you then undertake too much that you're not used to, you may well overstretch yourself."

GIVE YOURSELF A DAILY CHECK

□ Check yourself regularly for swollen hands, ankles, or feet, which would indicate a rise in blood pressure; also check for varicose veins and stiffness in the back, which might indicate that you are overdoing things.

□ Listen to your body. If something feels wrong or too strenuous, take a rest and try a different position. Again, don't do anything you didn't do before getting pregnant. If you suspect any problems or simply want to be reassured, consult your health practitioner.

SWIMMING

Swimming is good exercise in pregnancy because it keeps you buoyant and avoids putting pressure on your joints—and you won't feel self-conscious, since others can't see you in the water. Better still, for the first time in ages, you'll feel as light as a feather. An aqua-natal class is a great way to keep fit and supple for the whole nine months. Even if you can't swim, try exercising in the pool by holding onto the side with your back to the wall and cycling in the water, or by facing the side of the pool and swaying gently from side to side.

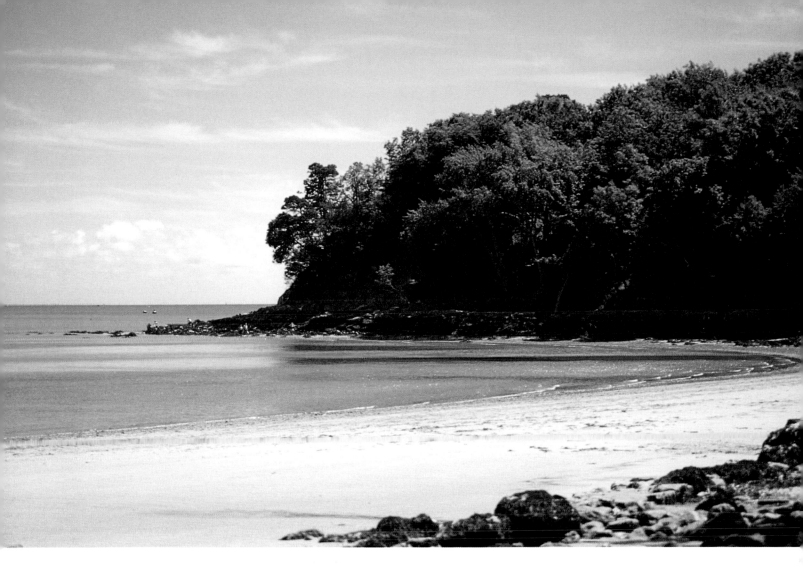

□ Buy a comfortable stretchy maternity swimsuit that will last throughout your pregnancy.

□ Always wash your hair after swimming to remove chlorine deposits, especially if it is blond or highlighted hair, which can turn brassy and yellow.

□ Apply a rich body cream after swimming or bathing, especially to your breasts and abdominal area.

□ Avoid jacuzzis, saunas, and steam rooms; they may be uncomfortably hot and raise a fetus's core temperature.

WALKING

Walking at a moderate pace is one of the best exercises in pregnancy. Don't struggle or get out of breath, but keep constantly moving. We all do this type of walking (to a greater or lesser extent) and have done since childhood, so there are no surprises in store. But air quality and a desirable destination both help to make walking more of a mission than a simple amble.

□ If you live in a city, take a break and a drive out of the city, away from traffic and pollution, to a place where the air you are breathing is good-quality air.

□ Wear proper trainers for comfort and for absorbing the shock as you pound the pavement.

□ Decide your walking route in advance. Give yourself plenty of time, especially as you get bigger. You may need to rest if you overexert yourself—and make sure you don't get stranded somewhere from which you can't get back without exerting yourself even more.

"I spent the whole nine months worrying. Everything from how I'd cope with a baby, would it be all right—and the birth itself worried me. I turned to Bach Flower Remedies, which I'd used in the past when flying, and they worked brilliantly for me."

SHEENA, MOTHER OF RUBY

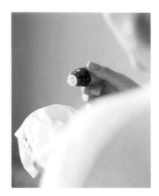

in pursuit of inner peace

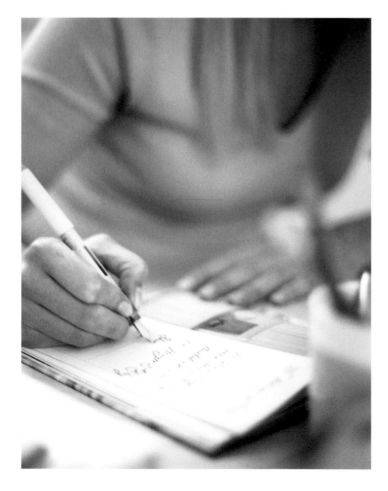

Keeping calm in pregnancy is crucial because a pregnant woman's anxiety can affect the fetus. Scientists at Columbia University in New York measured the anxiety rates of 32 pregnant women—determined by heart rate, blood pressure, and breathing rate—before, during, and after a psychological test designed to induce stress. The results showed a clear relationship between the women's anxiety levels and their babies' heart rates.

DON'T WORRY ABOUT A THING

Let's face it: pregnancy is an emotional rollercoaster. Just when you've peaked on the happiness barometer of life, you read something in the newspaper or watch a mildly sad video that you have seen a hundred times before—and suddenly you are in floods of tears.

In addition to the early physical changes that take place in pregnancy, which in themselves take time to get accustomed to, it is perfectly normal for a pregnant woman to experience mood swings as a result of the dramatic rise in levels of the hormones progesterone

there has never been a **better** time in your life to take advantage of **peaceful** quiet moments and **learn** some effective relaxation techniques

and estrogen during the first 14 weeks of pregnancy. If you also take into account the fact that you have only recently had your pregnancy confirmed (and may perhaps have been in denial), have felt at your worst (nausea), and may have had to keep the pregnancy hidden from your boss (more denial), the mood swings are not surprising. By about 14 weeks, they usually subside as your body adjusts to the pregnancy hormones, but many of us remain weepy and anxious at times throughout pregnancy.

While your body is in turmoil, there may be other, external reasons why you are experiencing mood swings. Choose a quiet moment to reflect on your thoughts and feelings. If you make a list of the things that are upsetting you and talk them through with your partner or a friend, it will help you to feel calmer.

You might be adjusting to the idea of becoming a mother and your changing image, or worrying about the baby itself—its health and future. Later in the pregnancy, mood swings may be caused by sheer panic as you start to think about labor, about what's ahead, and about all the things you won't be able to do so easily after the birth (such as be spontaneous).

EASY REMEDIES FOR STRESS

Exercise and aromatherapy are among the effective ways to reduce stress in pregnancy.

□ Exercise not only boosts circulation and strengthens muscles, but it also acts as a powerful aid to relaxation. However, as mentioned before, now is not the time to take up a new sport; stick to what you know and do everything in moderation. Even if you are unable or unwilling to follow a regular exercise routine, try to walk energetically for at least half an hour each day.

□ Add one drop of grapefruit essential oil to a clean handkerchief and inhale deeply three or four times to clear the mind. Do this whenever you feel tired, anxious, or unsure about things.

□ Balance your emotions and feel a little more in control of what's happening to you with Bach Flower Rescue Remedy, renowned for calming nerves and relieving anxiety. Four drops on the tongue or in a glass of water should help you unwind.

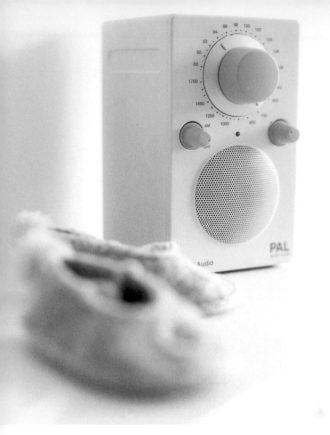

This is such an emotional time for you, and it's perfectly normal to feel anxious or tense. Learning how to cope with stress and tension will lead to a happier mom—and ultimately a happier baby, too.

1 Try this yoga position, which is very relaxing, good for the spine, and can accommodate a big tummy. Kneel on the floor, bend forward and stretch your arms out in front of you until your forehead rests on the floor. Breathe in and out slowly.

TEN WAYS TO... *keep calm*

2 Sit comfortably in a chair and lift your shoulders right up to your ears. Hold for a few seconds, then lower again. Repeat 3–4 times. Then to help free the neck, rock your head gently from side to side.

3 Why stand when you can sit? Why sit when you can lie down? Let this be your pregnancy mantra. Put your feet up and switch off as often as you can.

4 Lay back propped against a couple of cushions and keep yourself still, focusing only on your breathing, telling yourself that you feel warm and peaceful. Become aware of the weight of your body becoming heavier and heavier, limb by limb, until you feel unable to move. Concentrate on your breathing for five minutes, then when you are ready, wriggle your toes and fingers, open your eyes, and get up slowly.

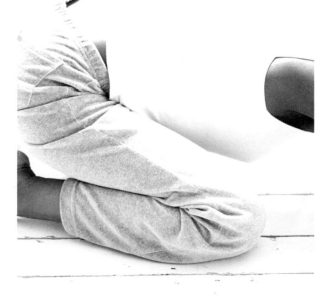

5 Bottle up this aromatherapy blend and keep it on hand so that, when you feel like it, you can massage it into pulse points: your wrists, the nape of your neck, and your temples. The blend consists of one drop of Roman chamomile and one drop of lavender essential oil in 10 ml (2 tsp) of sweet almond oil.

6 Sit cross-legged with your back supported by a sofa or chair. Close your eyes, and place one hand on your abdomen (below the ribs) and the other on your chest. Breathe in slowly through your nose, and concentrate on moving only the lower hand. Breathe quietly and calmly for 10 minutes.

7 We hold a lot of tension in the jaw without realizing it. Relax for a few moments and chew something slowly to relieve tension.

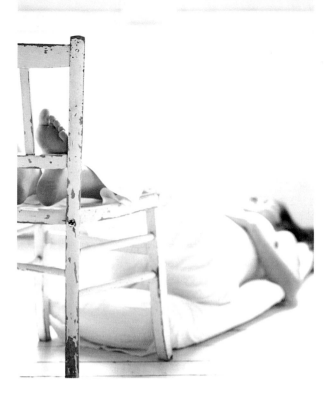

8 Listen to some classical music. One of my most pleasurable moments in pregnancy was to sit back in my favorite armchair listening to Mozart, breathing calmly (especially after a day at work) with one hand on my bump—especially once it started kicking. It helps you to focus on your baby and to relax and unwind; and the resonance of music played in pregnancy is believed to help develop your baby's brain.

9 Breathe in as slowly as you can (try to get to the count of ten), then breathe out equally slowly. It's a quick way to calm down, and it works.

10 Try a little calming aromatherapy. Place 2–3 drops of balancing geranium essential oil to a bowl with a little hot water. Put the bowl near a radiator or on a windowsill in the sunlight and leave the aroma to diffuse into the air. Use this time to practice any of your favorite breathing rituals mentioned here—combining two therapies into one, and making them both more effective.

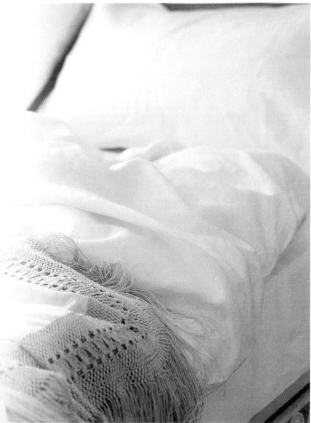

a good **balance** between work and **play**,
as well as lots of **rest**, will help you to **enjoy** your
pregnancy all the more

a life-changing experience

**With a baby on the way, there is no denying that the dynamics
between you and your partner will change—particularly when
you are about to adopt new roles within your home that will
probably transform the modern caring sharing relationship
that you may have worked hard to establish.**

TALKING TO YOUR PARTNER

No one teaches us to become parents. Hospitals have
prenatal classes labeled "parentcraft" or something
similar, but they are usually focused on the birth and
tell you little about being the parent, guardian, and
carer of a tiny dependent being.

Pregnancy can frequently bring couples closer than
they were before, enabling them to reach a new level
of caring and intimacy, and to share new visions and
plans for the future. But it is also easy to find that,
while your partner is being supportive to you, he may
well feel bewildered as well. Pregnancy is an emotional
rollercoaster for both of you. If he feels unable to give
you the help and encouragement you need, try to talk
about it together. For the moment, you have become
the main focus—perhaps he is finding it hard to adjust
to the shifting balance in your relationship.

Many expectant fathers suffer from bouts of anxiety,
but may be less able than the expectant mother to
recognize it in themselves. And in the early months, if
you are grappling with nausea and exhaustion, you
probably don't feel at all sexy, so he may feel physically
excluded without your even realizing it. It is easy to
assume that someone you know well understands—
but that is how misconceptions start. Whatever the
situation, discuss your thoughts and feelings, before
sensitivity turns into resentment.

ADAPTING YOUR LIFESTYLE

Establishing a good balance between work and play,
combined with masses of rest, will help you to get the
maximum amount of pleasure from your pregnancy.
□ Don't make huge demands on yourself. Imagine that
you have driven into the "slow lane" for a few months.
Everyone that matters will understand—if they don't,
who needs them? Pace yourself both at work and at
home. Don't say "yes" to everything. Delegate.
□ Consider rearranging your working day so that you
avoid traveling during rush hours. Perhaps you can work
from home one or two days a week?
□ When your body says relax—give in. Remind yourself
all the time to be kind to yourself.

"I was in denial—almost until the birth, if I'm honest—I went out and bought every book, because I didn't look or feel pregnant, and it only became real when I was able to look at it technically with pictures."

KATE, MOTHER OF EVIE

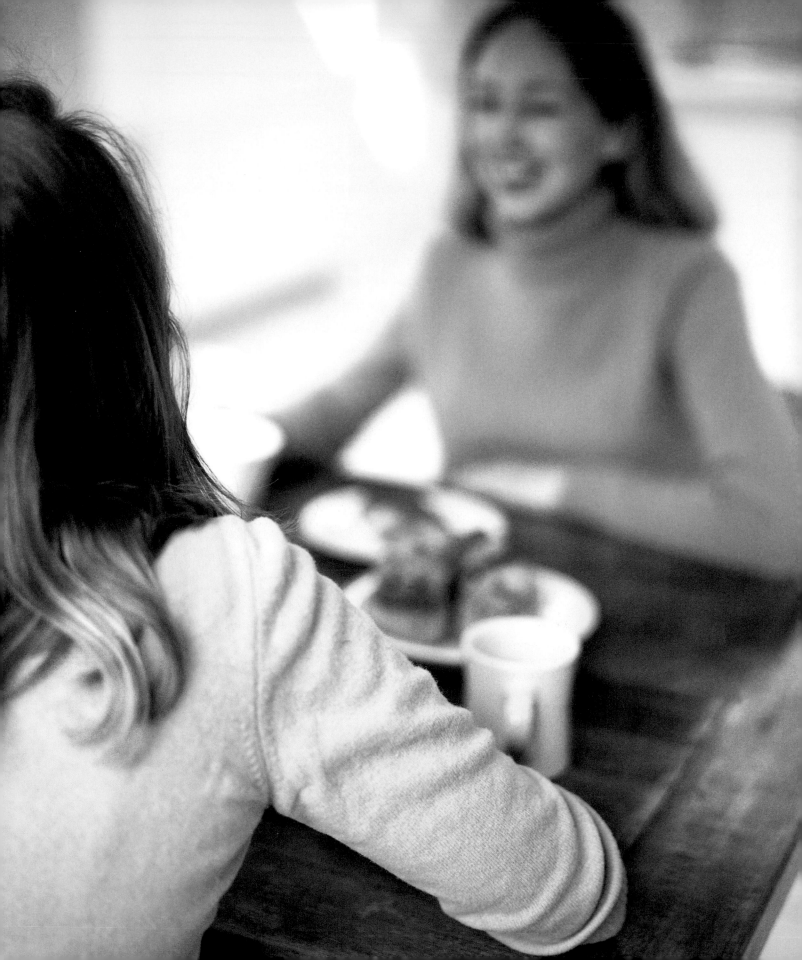

feeling good

This is your moment to shine. You have energy and vitality. You can't remember feeling this way before. You are blooming and gorgeous—and those who know you can see it. It feels good, and it does you good, too. Those hormones are surging, so keep on looking after yourself.

"I used to wear my long hair down all the time in pregnancy. It was so shiny—but it also helped to balance out my huge tummy and bottom."

HILARY, MOTHER OF JO

beautiful hair

At last those pregnancy hormones seem to have settled down and you have entered the stage when people often say, "You're blooming." The trials of early pregnancy, such as lank hair, greasy skin, and nausea, should now give way to a general feeling of wellbeing.

FEEDING YOUR HAIR

Is your hair thicker, shinier, and more manageable than it used to be? The theory is that the surge of estrogen in pregnancy encourages the hair to stay in place in its growing phase for longer than usual. The average life of a hair is four years, during which it grows uninterrupted before finally "resting" and falling out as new hairs emerge. In pregnancy, your hair, instead of falling out, stays put. So it not only looks thicker; it really is thicker.

Most women think their hair looks and feels its best during pregnancy. Those with fine or greasy hair notice the most dramatic difference because higher estrogen levels reduce the amount of oiliness on the scalp, so hair becomes less greasy, and fine hair looks thicker.

Vital vitamins and minerals for strong hair include:
□ Iron—found in meat, soy, yeast, wheat bran, and leafy green vegetables such as spinach.
□ B-group vitamins—found in wheatgerm, nuts, eggs, soy, and bananas.

□ Amino acids such as cysteine and methionine, the building blocks for keratin (the protein in hair and nails)—found in nuts, seeds, eggs, and meat.
□ Zinc—found in cheese (avoid unpasteurized soft cheese), brown rice, lentils, and oily fish such as sardine and mackerel.
□ Selenium—found in hard cheese, shrimp, and carrot.

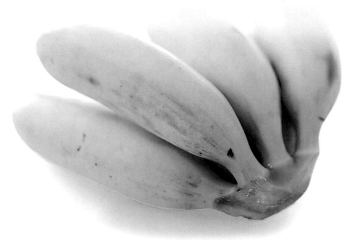

COLORING YOUR HAIR

There has been much controversy about whether or not hair dyes can harm unborn babies, but, according to leading trichologist Glen Lyons at the Phillip Kingsley Trichology Clinic in London, there is no evidence that they do. And, in pregnancy, anything that makes you feel good about yourself and builds your self-esteem will benefit your baby. But raised hormone levels may mean that the color takes more quickly than usual (and the shade may turn out differently, too), so go to a reputable and conscientious hairdresser—otherwise you may end up overprocessing your hair.

TEMPORARY HAIR LOSS

Well over 50 percent of new mothers suffer some hair loss after the birth. Most will notice that their hair looks much thinner than before they were pregnant, while others may lose big clumps of hair. This usually happens three to four months after the baby is born (although breastfeeding may delay it), but it is only temporary.

In pregnancy, the growing phase of the hair cycle has been extended so that each hair stays in place longer and you have more hair than usual. But after the birth, the "resting" phase in the cycle of hair growth and loss, which has been delayed, kicks in all at once—and suddenly the hair shedding that should have taken place over several months occurs almost overnight. Since no new hairs have had the chance to grow through, your hair suddenly looks much thinner.

The best way to make sure your hair grows back beautifully over the following 6 to 9 months is to eat a balanced diet rich in B vitamins, zinc, selenium, iron, and amino acids; breastfeeding mothers should make doubly sure they are eating well. If you boost your iron stores before, during, and after pregnancy, you stand a better chance of maintaining strong, healthy hair.

Once your hair starts to grow back, you may find that they stick up in all directions or form a "fringe" of baby hair. This may be a good moment to choose a short hairstyle that is easy to manage.

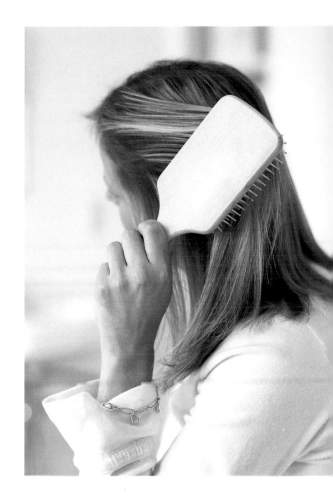

"When I had Felix, my hair came out in handfuls. Once it started growing back, I had new fluffy hairs that were hard to style. Friends recommended wax and spray gels to smooth the hairs down, and that helped me to cope until they got longer."

INGRID, MOTHER OF MAXIM AND FELIX

weeks 15–28 BEAUTIFUL HAIR

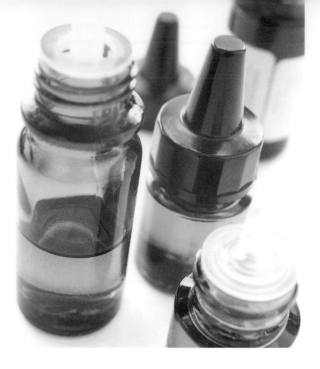

"Mandarin oil is a good oil to use in pregnancy—and it is safe to use throughout the nine months."

GLENDA TAYLOR, AROMATHERAPIST

pampering your skin

In the middle trimester of pregnancy, you are likely to feel better than ever in yourself—more energized, more focused: this is the time to reflect within and to pamper yourself from without.

CHANGES THAT AFFECT YOUR SKIN

At this stage of pregnancy, your body is in a beautiful period of energy. You can feel your baby moving—first as a flutter and progressively more responsive to your touch. Your shape is more pronounced and others, even strangers, respond to you in a positive way. At the same time, you may start to notice changes to your skin in response to the pregnancy.

□ Changes in skin pigmentation are evident on various parts of the body. The nipples and the areola usually darken, and freckles, moles, and birthmarks may become darker in color and bigger, so remember to use sun protection when you are outdoors.

□ Around the 16th week a dark vertical line called the "linea nigra" often appears down the center of the abdomen. It gets darker toward the end of the pregnancy but fades soon after the birth.

□ If the skin on your body becomes dry and sometimes itchy across the abdomen, add some nourishing oil to your bath water—try sweet almond or jojoba oil. If you do add oil to the bath, take extra care when you get in and out because it will make the bathtub slippery.

□ Sometimes a red skin rash called "intertrigo" occurs under the breasts or in the groin area. This is caused by excessive perspiration. If you develop intertrigo, wash and dry the area frequently, and use talcum powder to keep it dry. Soothe the skin with a cooling skin preparation such as calamine lotion, and wear loose cotton clothing in warm weather.

□ Many women develop stretch marks as their pregnancy progresses. These are caused by the skin becoming stretched beyond its normal elasticity as a result of the rapid weight gain and changes in hormone levels associated with pregnancy. Stretch marks begin as red indented lines around the breasts, thighs, and abdominal area, but will eventually fade to silvery streaks after a few months. However, nothing actually banishes stretch marks entirely.

Dry, pale Celtic skins suffer most from stretch marks, but they end up looking less noticeable on such a skin than on darker skins. Oilier olive skins tend to suffer from fewer marks, but they are more obvious, and the areas of the skin affected do not tan.

The best thing you can do to avoid stretch marks is to avoid putting on too much weight too quickly and keep the skin supple by regularly applying body oil or moisturizer after bathing. Professional anti-stretch-mark creams and lotions won't prevent or heal stretch marks—if your mother had them, the chances are that you will, too—but keeping your skin supple and soft may help to minimize their occurrence.

A REMEDY FOR STRETCH MARKS

"Mandarin oil is often used in aromatherapy skin treatments—helping to reduce scarring by encouraging skin-cell regeneration," says aromatherapist Glenda Taylor. Blend 2 drops of mandarin oil and 1 drop of lavender oil with 10 ml (2 tsp) of grapeseed or sweet almond oil and massage it into your abdominal area every evening before going to bed.

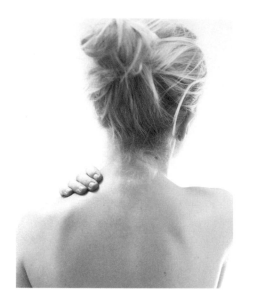

Midway through, this is your best chance to make the most of pregnancy. And when the bloom doesn't come naturally, cheat!

1 Exfoliate your skin. A gentle scrub twice a week, or once if your skin is feeling sensitive, will brighten up your complexion, even if you're feeling tired. Often, the simple ritual of caring for yourself—especially when you are not feeling quite yourself—can help to boost your mood and your senses and make you feel more energized and more positive inside and out.

TEN WAYS TO...*get the bloom*

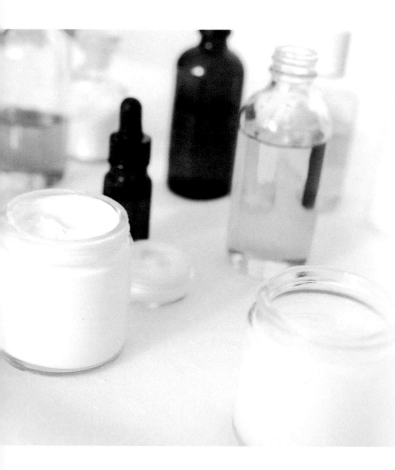

2 Use a revitalizing face cream containing vitamin C, which will help to brighten up dull, tired skin. In summer, you can simply substitute it for your usual moisturizer. In winter, or if your skin is especially dry, apply it underneath your usual face cream to boost your complexion.

3 Enhance your complexion by giving it a healthy vibrant glow. A light dusting of bronzing powder applied over the areas of your face and neck where you would naturally catch the sun—cheeks, temples, and collarbone—will instantly add a radiant gleam. Choose a bronzing powder that is neither matte nor glittery, but just slightly shimmery.

4 Alternatively, look for a cosmetic cream containing shimmery light-reflective particles. These are often golden or bronze, but when applied to the skin on the temples, cheekbones, browbones, and collarbone, they give a sheer, healthy-looking sheen to your skin—the make-up equivalent of radiance in pregnancy.

5 If you are not getting much sleep and are looking and feeling exhausted, try applying a small amount of lilac-colored matte powder underneath your eyes. Lilac will help to counteract any darkness in the area under the eyes and brighten up the way you look—even if you don't feel particularly bright.

6 A quick slick of lip balm over the lips keeps them looking natural and conditioned, but gives a hint of gloss, too. Stay with the natural look—or top up with your favorite lip color.

7 When your skin feels sensitive, make up a facial skincare blend to soothe minor irritations overnight. Mix 1 drop of lavender oil and 1 drop of Roman chamomile with 10 ml (2 tsp) of almond oil. Apply to clean skin and enjoy the aroma, which should help to send you to sleep.

8 Always carry around a refreshing facial spray. Whether it is an aromatherapy spray, a spray from your favorite skincare line, or simply water in an atomizer, a quick spritz to your skin helps to keep you cool and feeling fresh a great pick-me-up when you're fading at the end of a day at work.

9 Since your body temperature is raised during pregnancy, you may find that you perspire more than usual. Keep an antiperspirant deodorant on hand, or a tiny jar of sweetly perfumed, shimmery, seductive body powder to absorb excess oils.

10 If flawless skin is not an element of your pregnancy, choose a cream-to-powder foundation that glides onto your skin and covers spots and blemishes really well without making you feel as if you're wearing loads of makeup. It is easy to apply, looks natural—and you can touch it up throughout the day, too, without making your makeup look heavy.

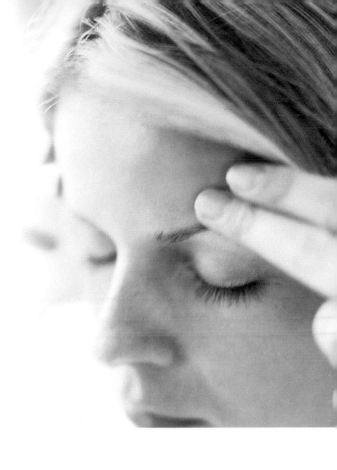

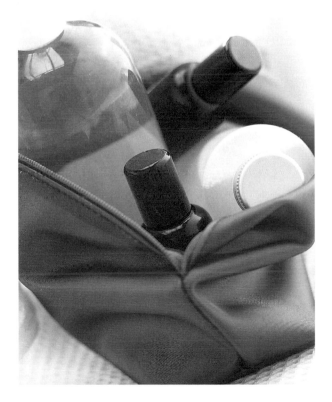

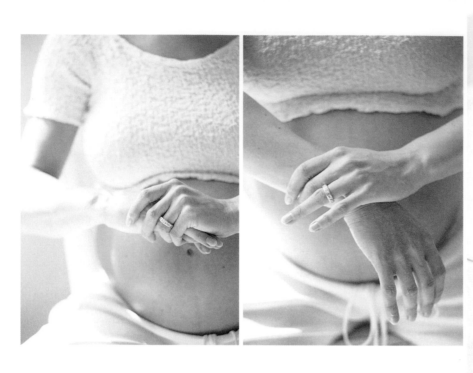

treats for hands and feet

Even though the focus right now is on your expanding waistline, you can draw attention to other parts of your body with a little extra self-love. If they are pampered, creamed, and polished, your hands and feet will help you to look and feel more nurtured and groomed.

HAND CARE

Your hands are likely to be immersed in more hot water than ever before while you are caring for a young baby. So now is the perfect time to create a mini-pampering ritual for your hands.

Keep a tube of your favorite hand cream by every sink in your house, one by your bed, and one in the car. Reapply at every opportunity: when you get up and when you go to bed, immediately after washing your hands, before you drive, or after you've parked.

MASSAGING YOUR HANDS

This do-it-yourself hand massage takes minutes.

□ Apply a little hand cream.

□ Relax your hands by squeezing them. Place one hand over the other and gently but firmly squeeze all over, then swap hands and repeat with the other hand.

□ Gently flick and shake your hands from the wrists.

□ Hold your hands out in front of you. Take the thumb of your right hand and place it in the palm of your left hand, then support your left hand using your right palm. Use short, sliding movements with your thumb (called "petrissage" in massage terminology) to help stretch and relax your hands. Do this for 3 to 5 minutes, then swap hands and repeat.

A FRENCH MANICURE

The best way to achieve neat, polished, natural-looking nails is to give yourself a French manicure.

□ Apply a clear base-coat over clean nails.

□ Paint white polish over the natural white tips of your nails to make them look whiter, healthier, and more defined. If you make a mistake, take a small artist's paint brush, dip it into nail-polish remover, and smooth away the error.

□ By the time you have finished your last nail, the first should be dry, so paint one coat of pale pink polish over the entire nail, including the tip.

□ Finish with a final top-coat to seal all your hard work. Allow 30 minutes to dry.

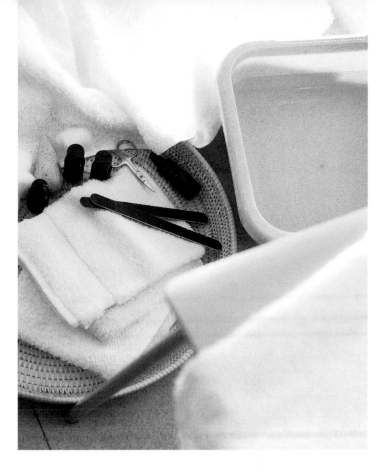

FOOT CARE

The golden rule for feet that always look good is to keep a jar of foot cream by your bed and religiously massage it into your feet before you go to sleep each night. Nighttime is the only time when our feet are free from the stress and strain of bearing our bodies around—and, with the extra burden you are carrying, you have even more reason to pamper your feet.

To keep your feet healthy in pregnancy, treat them two or three times a week to the following routine.

□ Buff any hard skin on the soles of your feet before soaking them—otherwise, you may remove more skin than is comfortable, which will make your heels tender. A long foot file is especially useful—as your pregnancy progresses, you will find it harder and harder to reach your toes properly.

□ Cut your toenails straight across using nail scissors. Never use nail clippers; they are frequently curved and do not cut correctly, encouraging the toenail to split or an ingrowing toenail to develop.

□ Use your normal body exfoliator on your feet and massage it in well for softer, smoother feet. Pay particular attention to the areas around the toes and the cuticles, where skin tends to become dry and flaky, making your feet look less pampered and cared for.

□ Add 3 drops of lemon oil to fresh water for a refreshing antiseptic and antibacterial soak.

□ Pat your feet dry and apply a little cuticle remover to the cuticles around the base of each toenail. Leave the cuticle remover on for 1 or 2 minutes, then remove it using a clean cotton swab, pressing down firmly on the nail and rubbing away as much old cuticle from the nail as possible.

□ Finish by applying plenty of moisturizer to your feet. It makes a dramatic difference, and just this one bit of daily attention quickly improves their appearance.

□ Polish your feet off. Wipe the nails clean, making sure that they are free from any cream, so that you can apply nail polish smoothly without streaking.

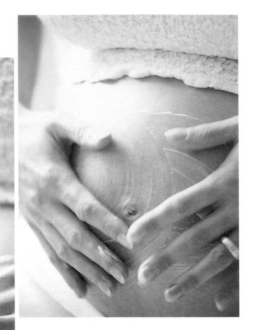

> "I massaged in plenty of Clarins Tonic Oil from the moment I discovered I was pregnant. I didn't get a single stretch mark until I had my third child."
>
> **KATE, MOTHER OF ELLIOTT, EDWARD AND MILES**

the big tummy massage

Think of the big tummy massage as both a treat and a treatment. It is a treat for you and your growing baby, too, encouraging early bonding, and it is a treatment for your body—to help prevent stretch marks.

A THERAPEUTIC EXPERIENCE

Touch is a vital part of human existence. To be touched, caressed, and stroked by a loved one is a therapeutic experience in itself—and, for a pregnant woman in labor, it certainly helps to feel comfortable in response to your birthing partner's touch.

Equally, in pregnancy, you can enjoy a deep sense of relaxation by touching and massaging your own abdominal area. And you will soon start to feel a special closeness with your baby, too.

Before beginning the massage, make sure you have available a copious amount of a rich oil or cream, such as wheatgerm, jojoba, or sweet almond—a preparation that will give a smooth massage and help improve the texture and tone of your skin. Each movement in this massage is slow and soothing, and slides across the skin, with lots of repetitions to allow the oil to penetrate fully and nourish your skin as much as possible.

PREPARING FOR THE MASSAGE

The best position for the massage in the middle months is lying on your back propped up by three pillows, so you are half-sitting. (Nearer full term, you may prefer to lie on your side with your knees bent.) Take care never to press down on the tummy area during any strokes. Keep all movements as light and gentle as a caress.

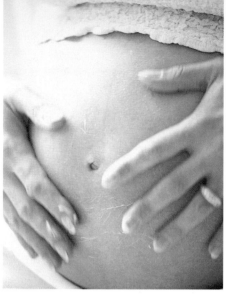
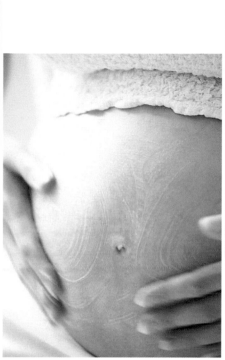
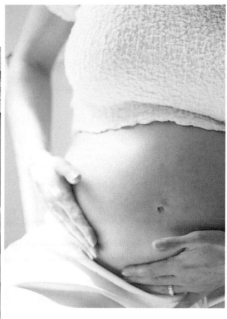

in addition to **helping** prevent stretch marks, a tummy massage will encourage you to **relax** and allow you to establish early **bonding** with your baby through **loving** strokes

STEP BY STEP

Warm the oil or cream between your hands before applying it to your abdominal area.

□ Start by taking one hand and gently warming your tummy with small, circular massage movements in a clockwise direction. Continue doing this for 3 to 5 minutes, making the circular movements gradually wider and wider across the tummy.

□ Place your hands, palms down, at the base of the ribs over the solar plexus, with your fingers pointing up to the chest. Draw your hands out to the sides, then pull them down the waist more firmly but gently around over the hips, stopping just below the navel. Continue doing this movement for 3 to 5 minutes.

□ Next, do a firm sidestroke up the waist. Place both hands, palms down, against the top of one thigh, with the fingers as far around as is comfortable. Then slide your hands up the sides of your torso, one after the other in a slow flowing stroke. Work from the thigh up to the base of the ribs for 3 to 5 minutes. Repeat on the other side for 3 to 5 minutes.

□ Finish by gently massaging the tummy again. Make large sweeping circles as if you were writing a big "e" on your tummy—always in a clockwise direction.

> "Rosewood essential oil is from the woods. It has its roots in the earth and is very grounding and mothering."
>
> **NOELLA GABRIEL, AROMATHERAPIST AND MOTHER OF KATE**

aromatherapy in pregnancy

This powerful aromatic mood therapy using essential oils from plants can be very beneficial during pregnancy. You can use key safe aromatherapy oils to relax and calm you down at times of greatly heightened emotion.

DECIDING WHICH OILS TO USE

Aromatherapy (using the scent of essential oils for healing) offers the perfect mood-enhancing antidote to stress, anxiety, insomnia, and discomfort in pregnancy. But opinion about which, if any, oils to use varies from one aromatherapist to another, and from one book to another—if only because the training and experience in this field varies almost as much as the effects that essential oils can have on your body.

Leading aromatherapist Glenda Taylor, a trusted friend of mine, says that, in her experience, "As long as you read the labels, use a little common sense, and do not abuse the oils, essential oils can be absolutely invaluable during pregnancy. They are nowhere near as potentially damaging as many foods and drinks we ingest at this sensitive time—such as coffee."

As a rule, a number of relaxing, calming oils (listed here) are considered safe during pregnancy provided that—as with anything in pregnancy—you are careful to follow any instructions or advice given and never to overdo it. (All reputable manufacturers state on the product label when an essential oil should not be used in pregnancy.) Avoid any highly stimulating, highly sedative oils, or emmenagogue oils (which stimulate menstruation), or oxytocic oils (which stimulate contractions and may induce labor).

If you plan to use aromatherapy in pregnancy—and I recommend that you do, to achieve a more serene state of mind and body—refer to the list of oils for each stage of pregnancy compiled by Glenda (see opposite page). The oils listed are by no means all the oils you could use, but they neither stimulate nor sedate the systems of the body to any great extent.

Citrus oils are beneficial, but since the skin is more sensitive during pregnancy, orange and lemon may itch, though will not do harm—they are great in a diffuser. Grapefruit and lime are excellent, as are mandarin and tangerine.

first trimester

Mandarin, tangerine, rosewood, and howood (an oil that you may prefer to use instead of rosewood, which is an endangered species), plus any citrus oil (lemon, grapefruit, or orange) in a diffuser.

second trimester

All the above oils, plus elemi, lemongrass, frankincense, neroli, palmarosa, petitgrain, and sandalwood.

third trimester

Lavender and rose essential oils can be used after the sixth month of pregnancy, and chamomile oil can also be added to the list. Try using rose in place of sandalwood in the Relax Blend, and lavender in place of palmarosa or lemongrass in the Balance Blend (see below).

postnatal

After the birth, in addition to the oils listed here, you can use bergamot and jasmine oils to combat feelings of depression, fennel oil also eases nervous tension and stimulates milk production in breastfeeding mothers.

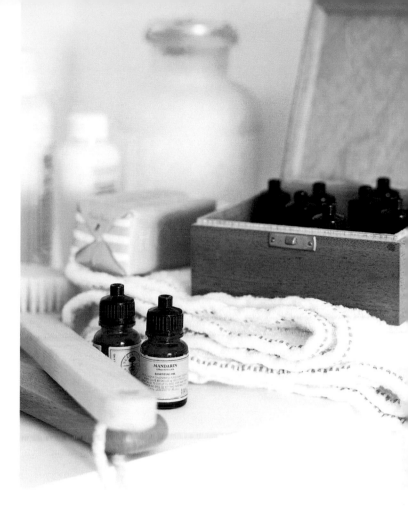

MAKE YOUR OWN PREGNANCY BLENDS

There is a choice of carrier oils that can be blended together for their various therapeutic effects—some are, for example, richer, lighter, or more antioxidant than others. Popular favorites include jojoba, almond, peach kernel, apricot, and vitamin E oils. If you can't get hold of vitamin E oil, you can simply break open a few vitamin E capsules. (Please note that 10 ml is equivalent to 2 teaspoons; 5 ml is equivalent to 1 teaspoon.)

The carrier oils included in the blends described on this page can be replaced by 30 ml (6 tsp) of base cream or lotion, using the same amount of essential oil. (Creams and lotions take less essential oil per milliliter.) If you down that route, you can still add a few drops of the carrier oils if you would like to increase the moisturizing and nourishing qualities of the blend.

If you are in any doubt about your state of health, which oils to use, or how much, it is crucial to consult a qualified aromatherapist to set your mind at ease.

relax blend

Mix 10 ml almond oil with 5 ml jojoba oil and add:

3 drops mandarin

3 drops neroli

1 drop sandalwood

revive blend

Mix 10 ml apricot oil with 5 ml rosehip oil and add:

3 drops grapefruit

2 drops petitgrain

2 drops rosewood

balance blend

Mix 10 ml peach kernel oil with 5 ml vitamin E oil and add:

5 drops sandalwood

1 drop palmarosa

1 drop lemongrass

if you can **tune** in to your **body**, it will help you to **feel** more **intuitive** about **niggling** aches and pains

"With each of my babies I had the early CVS test at
11 weeks. There is a family history of cystic fibrosis,
and I felt the risk of miscarriage (1 in 50) far
outweighed the pain of such an illness. Each time
was worse than the one before—we knew what we
had to lose. But we were incredibly blessed with
each child, and they're all healthy."

JO, MOTHER OF OLIVIA, WILLIAM, AND PHOEBE

staying well

**It is easy to become overanxious about
your pregnancy—especially if you have
experienced a previous miscarriage or had
difficulty conceiving. If this is your first
child, the anxiety may stem quite simply
from the fact that you feel a complete
novice, unsure about many things. Try to
tune in to your body, so that you can react
more intuitively to physical developments.**

WHEN TO SEEK MEDICAL ADVICE

If you feel at all concerned about anything relating to
your pregnancy, consult your health practitioner—they
are there to help and reassure you. Remember that
you are individual, and each pregnancy is individual.
What one woman experiences may or may not happen
to another. But even the "normal" changes that take
place in pregnancy may seem worrying or alarming
when experienced for the first time.

Don't forget to attend your prenatal checkups. These
are designed to monitor your health and the progress
of your pregnancy and to make sure any problem is

detected early. Seek medical advice if you experience
any of the following:

☐ Vaginal bleeding.

☐ Abdominal cramps or pains that get worse.

☐ Severe headaches, dizziness, nausea, blurred vision,
and/or swollen ankles or feet; these symptoms could
indicate pre-eclampsia, which affects one in ten
pregnancies.

☐ High temperature, fever symptoms, or any other
symptoms that worry you.

SPECIAL TESTS

If you are particularly concerned about the health of
your baby, you may want to arrange for a fetal test
such as CVS (chorionic villus sampling), amniocentesis,
cordocentesis, or a nuchal fold test. You are only
expected to have these tests if your risks are higher
than average—that is, you are over the age of 35 or
are aware of a genetic disorder in your family—and if
you are prepared to terminate your pregnancy should
the result detect some abnormality. However, these
tests can also provide reassurance, which may be what
you need if you are overanxious.

super energy foods

Whether you are pregnant or not, eating well—attending to quality rather than quantity—will automatically boost your energy levels. Good nutrition at this time means that your baby will not have to feed off you. However, if your hair and nails are looking weak, or your skin has failed to improve, it may be a sign that your diet is not leaving enough nutrients for you. Listen to your body. Give in to cravings—they indicate a need. If it is something sugary that you desire, make sure you balance it out with plenty of good wholefoods.

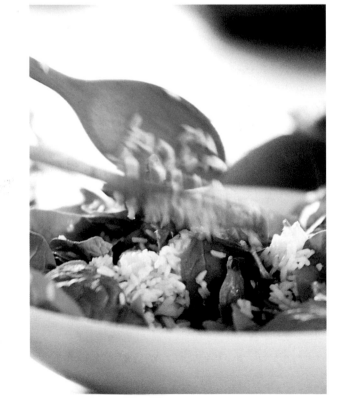

THE ELEMENTS OF GOOD NUTRITION

When you are pregnant, you are not only feeding yourself and your developing baby from within, you are also feeding the placenta.

Vital vitamins and minerals should come mainly from food, since it can be difficult to gauge for yourself which supplements to take in pregnancy, or how much of a particular supplement it is advisable to take— certain vitamins such as vitamin A can be toxic if taken in excess. That is why it is essential to maintain a well-balanced diet full of vitamin- and mineral-rich wholefoods (unprocessed foods that are readily available in their natural state) that can be eaten either raw or lightly cooked.

Vitamins and minerals—including iron, calcium, magnesium, and zinc—are important in pregnancy because they help stimulate your body's natural mechanisms, preventing problems such as cramps, fluid retention, and high blood pressure, promoting instead healthy blood flow and good circulation.

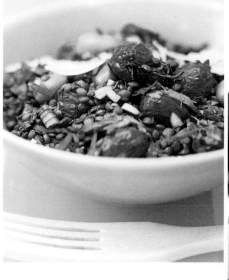
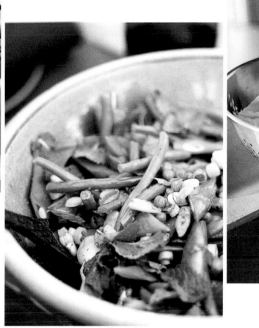
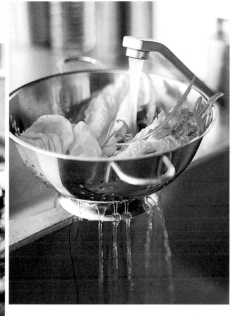

A DIET FOR ENERGY

To maintain a high level of energy in pregnancy, make sure that your diet includes the following.

□ Fish (especially oily fish for Omega-3 and Omega 6 essential fatty acids).

□ Freshly made soup.

□ Poultry.

□ Free-range eggs three times a week.

□ Plenty of fresh colored vegetables and green leafy salads.

□ Fresh fruit.

□ Legumes, such as garbanzo beans and lentils.

□ Nuts and seeds. (Eating peanuts in pregnancy is not believed to cause peanut allergy in the baby, but some mothers prefer to be cautious and avoid them at this time.)

□ Granola and oatmeal.

□ Soy beans and tofu.

□ Olive oil and flaxseed oil.

□ Minimal quantities of sugar.

DRINK MORE WATER

All pregnant women need plenty of water. It is a misconception that, if you suffer from fluid retention in pregnancy, you should cut back on your fluid intake. The opposite is the case. If you increase the amount of water you drink (up to eight glasses a day); it will flush the kidneys through and help to alleviate the condition.

ENERGY EATING RITUALS

□ Drink flower and fruit teas instead of coffee and tea.

□ Don't eat when you are upset or angry.

□ To aid digestion, eat slowly and while seated.

□ Don't drink while you eat—otherwise, it dilutes your digestive enzymes, leading to poor digestion.

□ Don't go any longer than 2½ hours without food.

□ Make sure you eat a nutritious breakfast to fuel your low blood sugar level first thing in the morning.

□ Buy organic where possible. Pesticide residues are linked to a growing number of allergies in young children. Start as you mean to go on.

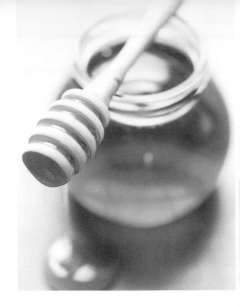

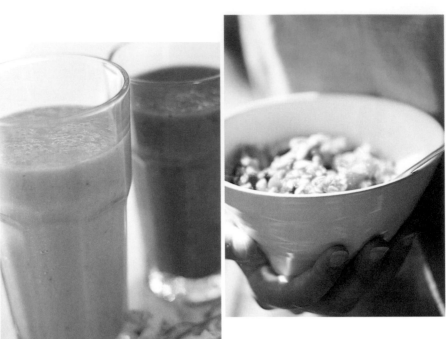

GETTING OFF TO A GOOD START

Every morning, make a pitcher full of a delicious fresh fruit smoothie that you can drink through the day. It is not only a healthy drink that helps to curb those blood sugar lows—it is also a great way to get extra antioxidant vitamins and calcium into your body. All you need is a blender, a choice of fruit, a dairy or soy base, a few chunks of ice, and a scoop of ice cream for a little extra indulgence. Try one of the blends listed below.

POWER SNACKS

Some fruits are particularly beneficial in pregnancy.

□ Avocado contains essential B vitamins and vitamin E, plus copper for red blood cells and iron absorption.

□ Banana contains high levels of B6, and is rich in potassium, which helps to balance your blood pressure.

□ Citrus fruits are full of antioxidant vitamins, vital for collagen formation, and folic acid, which increases the amount of oxygen carried around your body.

berry delicious blend

8 strawberries

1 large banana

1 cup (250 g) blueberries

1½ pints (800 g) natural bio-yogurt

sweet-natured blend

6 kiwi fruit

¾ cup (150 g) fresh cherries (stoned)

1 cup (200 g) white seedless grapes

1½ pints (800 g) natural bio-yogurt

highly exotic blend

10 passionfruit (strained)

1 large pineapple

4 bananas

1½ pints (800 g) natural bio-yogurt

blooming gorgeous blend

1 pineapple

2 mangoes

3 bananas

2 cans coconut milk

peach, pear, and plum blend

1 apple

2 peaches

3 pears

10 plums

1½ pints (800 g) natural bio-yogurt

3 tbsn clear honey

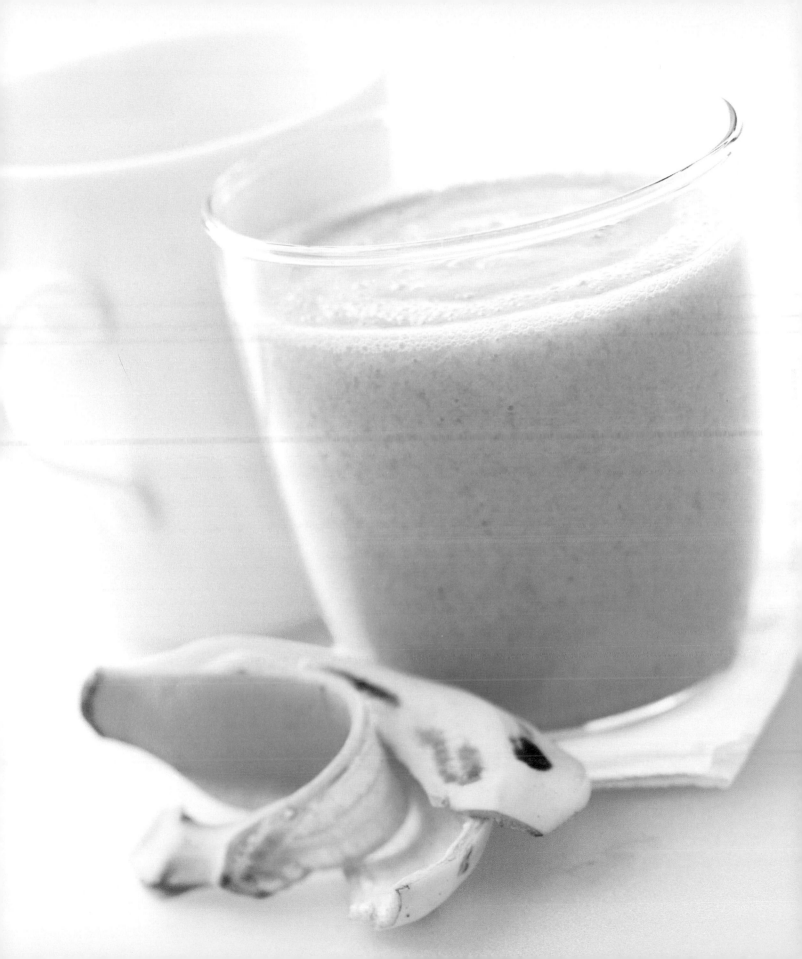

> "I can honestly say that if I knew then (with baby number one) what I know now (after baby number three), I'd have listened more attentively the first time around."

JO, MOTHER OF OLIVIA, WILLIAM, AND PHOEBE

exercising your pelvic floor

If there is one thing you really should do for yourself in pregnancy, it is to exercise your pelvic floor. Every gynecologist, obstetrician, physiotherapist, and urologist would agree. Apart from helping prevent stress incontinence, the exercises will encourage healing and recovery in the pelvic area after the birth.

WHAT IS THE PELVIC FLOOR?

The pelvic floor is a common term for the muscular "sling" in the base of the pelvis that supports your bladder, vagina, and bowel. And it is your pelvic floor that bears the increasing weight of your uterus and your baby as it grows, and which takes the strain of the baby's head in preparation for birth. Cough, and you will feel where it is.

As is the case with any muscles, good tone and support enable them to spring back into shape easily after use, but without exercise the muscles of the pelvic floor become weak, leading to urinary stress incontinence—a condition that is estimated to affect two-thirds of new mothers.

HOW TO EXERCISE

□ First, locate your pelvic-floor muscles. If you cough once or twice, you can sense where they are.

□ Now, breathing normally, practice slowly pulling up the muscles between your legs (without using your leg, abdominal, or buttock muscles) and holding them for a moment before slowly releasing them again. Repeat ten times in a row. Try to remember to do this as often as you can throughout the day.

TAKING THE ELEVATOR TO THE PENTHOUSE

A tip for exercising your pelvic-floor muscles is offered by physiotherapists at Queen Charlotte's & Chelsea Hospital in London. They recommend imagining that your pelvic floor is an elevator going up five floors. As you tighten the muscles, imagine you have stopped at the second floor, pause, then tighten again to reach the third floor, pause, then tighten again for the fourth— and so on until you get to the top floor. Work up to the penthouse if you can! Then practice stopping off at each floor on the way down as you release the muscles.

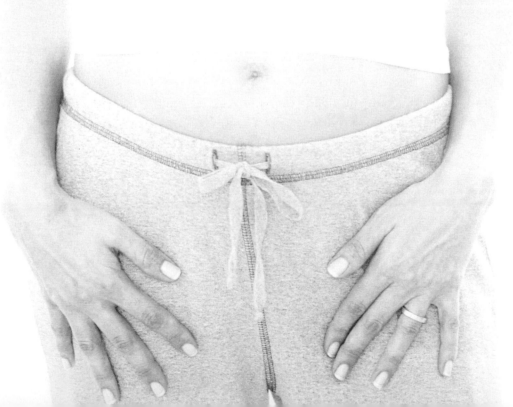

imagine that your **pelvic** floor is an elevator going up five floors; to make sure you are **exercising** it efficiently, **you** need to **tighten** it between each level

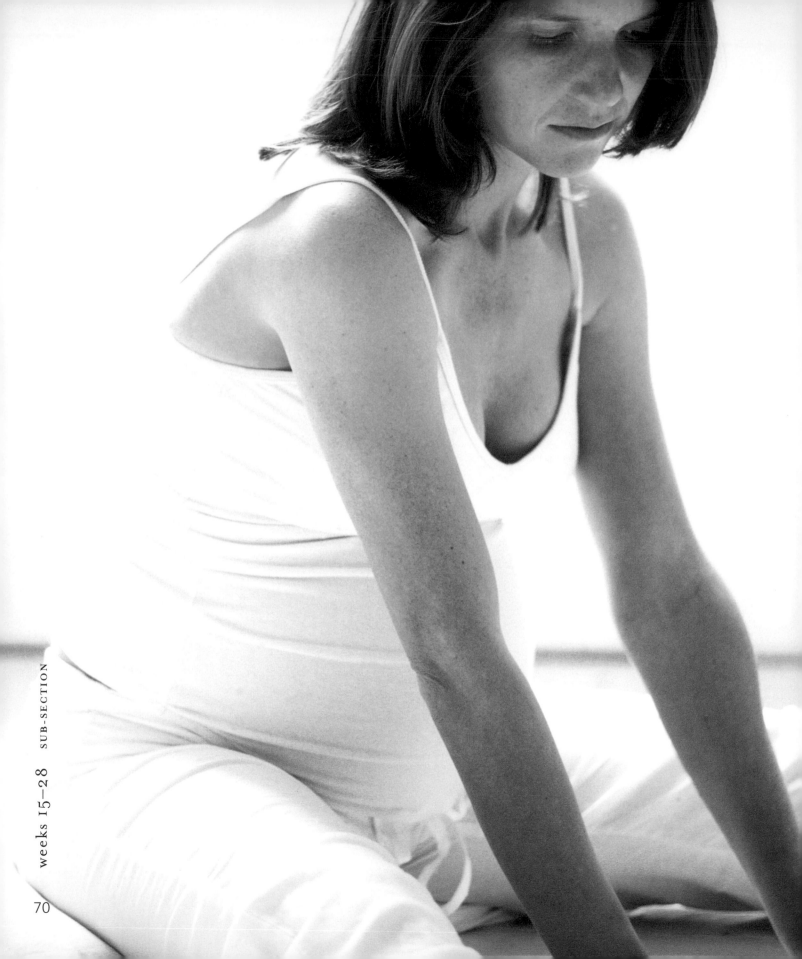

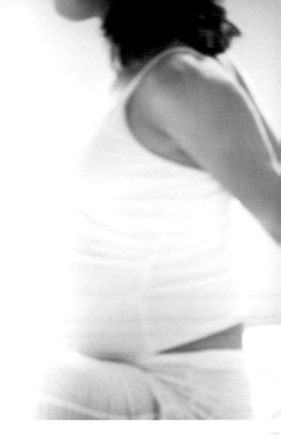

stretching and toning

Exercising to keep your body supple, stretched, and toned is vital in pregnancy. You want to know—and feel—that you are the fittest you can be at this important time. The yoga moves described on the following pages, all of which involve slow, gentle stretching, are easy to do at home and will help you to keep your body in perfect shape.

THE GROUND RULES

This section covers five yoga exercises that you can do at home: the Seat, the Shrug, the Squat, the Lunge, and the Cat (see pages 72–73). Take care never to strain or overstretch yourself when exercising in pregnancy. Do all exercises slowly and with care. If you have a history of miscarriage or are having any difficulties with this pregnancy, check with your doctor or midwife before undertaking any exercise, particularly in the first three months. Other points to remember are:

❑ Keep breathing deeply at a steady, controlled pace throughout the exercise session.

❑ Avoid sit-ups or raising both legs simultaneously since this can affect the abdominal muscles.

❑ Always get up from the floor by rolling onto your side and using your arms to push you up.

MAKE YOURSELF COMFORTABLE

Before embarking on any floor exercises in pregnancy, it is worth equipping yourself with the right accessories to make the experience comfortable and enjoyable.

❑ Buy extra pillows. You can use them under your knees to give your back support during some exercises, and to raise your head when lying on the floor. They are also useful when your sleep is interrupted—to support your knees and back for extra comfort. And, after your baby is born, you can put a spare pillow on your lap to raise the baby to the right level for breastfeeding.

❑ Get yourself a big, stylish beanbag. Now often used as an alternative to the rigid couch in pregnancy by the holistic company Elemis, a beanbag is unmatched for comfort during pregnancy. "So many pregnancy 'treatments' try to squeeze you into a variety of holes on a couch," says Noella Gabriel of Elemis. "A beanbag has the ability to mold with your ever-expanding body, bust, and bump in a comforting and dignified way—whether you're three or nine months gone."

❑ Sit on it, lay on it, rock and roll on it: look for a big inflatable ball that, when used like a beanbag, can help to relieve backache, relax mother and baby, and give support in specific pelvic exercises throughout pregnancy, labor, and birth.

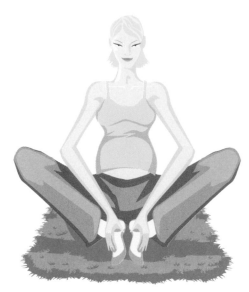

THE SEAT

The Seat strengthens the back and makes the thighs and pelvis more flexible—a great asset in childbirth. Sit on the floor with your back straight and the soles of your feet together. Hold your ankles and keep your heels as close to your body as possible. Your elbows should rest comfortably on your thighs. Use your elbows to press your thighs down toward the floor to increase the stretch. Breathe in; breathe out fully while you stretch. Hold for a count of ten, breathing deeply. Repeat ten times. If it feels difficult, do one knee at a time.

THE SHRUG

The Shrug releases tension in the neck and shoulders, and strengthens the upper back and arm muscles. Sit upright on the edge of a chair with your back straight and knees at right angles to the floor, arms straight down. Looking ahead, breathe in and shrug your shoulders tightly. Breathe out as your shoulders go down, then pull your arms back behind you, shoulders relaxed and straight, so that the backs of your hands are facing forward. Breathe in to return to the original position. Repeat ten times.

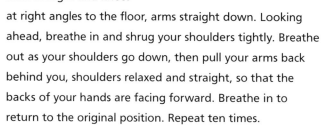

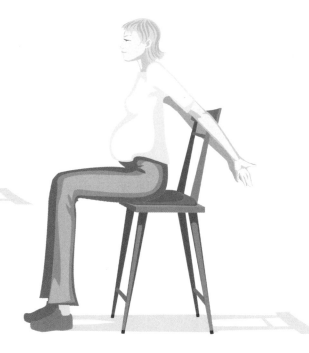

everyone says **"rest"**—but a certain amount of **activity** is necessary; remember that **exercise** gives you energy, so even at the **slowest pace**, it is better than doing nothing

THE SQUAT

The Squat makes the pelvic joints more flexible and helps to strengthen the back and thigh muscles. Use a chair for support until you feel able to do without it. Stand facing the chair with feet hip-width apart, feet turned slightly outward. Keeping your back straight and your heels to the ground, breathe in, and breathe out as you squat low. Stay like this for as long as it is comfortable. Get up slowly to avoid feeling dizzy. Repeat three times.

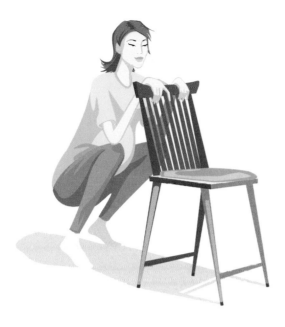

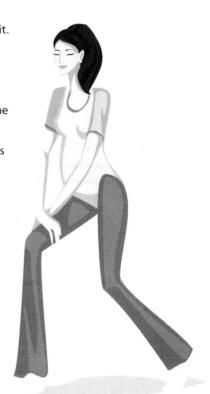

THE LUNGE

The Lunge strengthens the legs and improves the posture. Stand upright, back straight, tummy held in (as far as possible). Breathe in, and as you breath out, take a step forward with one leg, supporting yourself with your hands on your outward thigh. Keep your back leg slightly bent, and your heel as close to the ground as you can to increase the stretch.

THE CAT

The Cat stretches the spine from head to tail and strengthens the abdominal muscles without strain. Kneel on all fours, with your hands and knees a short distance apart, and breathe in. As you release the breath, gently arch your back, pushing your head down so you feel a complete stretch. Breathe in as you bring your head up. Breathe out and relax. Repeat ten times.

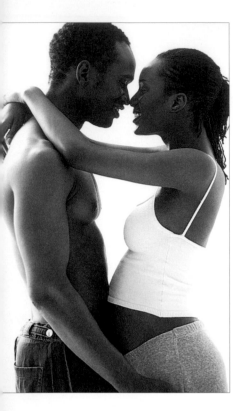

"I feel even more sexy when I'm pregnant – hence the reason I keep having babies. I think it's partly because I'm naturally thin and suddenly I become more rounded and curvaceous and my breasts are so much bigger. I love it and so does my husband."

HELEN, MOTHER OF ELLIOTT, EDWARD, AND MILES

in the mood for love

In the second, "vitality" trimester, you may find that you are feeling more amorous than before—but there are no guarantees!

REDISCOVERING YOUR SEXUALITY .
During the fifth and sixth months of pregnancy, the pregnant woman's blood supply and vaginal secretions increase—which is why many women find themselves more aware of their sexuality again in the middle of the second trimester. However, some couples find that their desire fluctuates throughout the pregnancy, and declines as the birth approaches.

Partners sometimes worry that they will "hurt the baby" during sex, but comfortable intercourse positions that neither press on your tummy nor involve deep penetration are considered safe. Feeling positive about

your rounded pregnant body is important to your overall sense of wellbeing and obviously has an effect on how alluring you feel. Your partner may or may not be keen to continue having sex during pregnancy.

Make sure you talk to each other about your feelings and needs. This is a very intimate time together, and one that should be enjoyed rather than endured.

WHEN TO AVOID MAKING LOVE
Avoid sex in pregnancy in the following circumstances:
□ You have a history of miscarriage in the early months of pregnancy.
□ You have a history of premature labor.
□ Bleeding occurs in pregnancy.
□ You or your partner has an infection or pelvic pain.
□ The waters break or you are leaking amniotic fluid.
□ The cervix is dilated.

TIME FOR TOGETHERNESS

You can put yourself and your partner in the mood for love with a little something to stimulate the senses.

□ Slip into a bath for two containing a soothing blend of essential oils that he, too, will enjoy—for example, 2 drops each of sandalwood, frankincense, and mandarin oils.

□ Create the perfect sultry and erotic environment by lighting a candle and scenting the air with calming sandalwood from a diffuser.

□ Flaunt it—and that means all of it! Powder yourself with a shimmery seductive body powder.

□ Massage in a little extra body-conditioning oil. You are not only doing your body a favor; it will give your skin a sexy, baby-soft sheen to make you irresistible.

□ You can still wear sexy lingerie, but don't buy it just for the pregnancy. Look for all-in-one, super-stretch bodysuits with lace trim, which not only look pretty, but also manage to hold you together and give the bump extra support after six months.

□ Listen to resonant classical music that will relax all three of you at the same time.

LOVE BLEND IN PREGNANCY

Prepare the following pregnancy Love Blend created by aromatherapist Glenda Taylor. Keep using it after pregnancy to help to counteract stretch marks—and baby number two won't be too far behind.

Combine 10 ml (2 tsp) almond oil with 5 ml (1 tsp) jojoba oil to make a carrier oil. Add 3 drops each of mandarin and neroli oils and 1 drop of sandalwood oil to the carrier. Ask your partner to massage the oil gently into the nape of your neck as well as into your shoulders, hands, legs, feet, and bump.

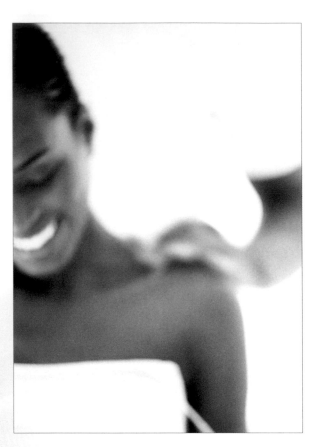

the loving touch

Touch is the tender way to communicate. I know that I could never have survived my three pregnancies as well as I did without wonderful intuitive, relaxing massages from my husband. Partners: please read this section and take special note.

THE BENEFITS OF MASSAGE

Whether you are pregnant or not, regular massage is beneficial to both mind and body. But pregnancy is an excellent time to ask your partner to practice a few wonderful strokes because massage relaxes, calms, and soothes in next to no time, as well as helping to relieve various aches and pains. It can also prove extremely beneficial during the early stages of labor. For that reason, these massage guidelines are addressed to your own personal amateur masseur.

FOOT MASSAGE

Rub a little oil into the palms of your hands, then pick up one of her feet and rest it on your thigh, sole facing up. Gently stroke the entire sole using flat hands, keeping your fingers together. Then make a fist and very gently knead the sole of her foot from the heel to the toes. Gently massage each toe individually and finish by sandwiching her foot between the palms of your hands and sweep from the heel to the toes. Repeat with her other foot.

BACK MASSAGE

Sit her comfortably in an armless chair so that she faces toward the back of it. Oil your hands and spread them over the skin on her back with light, sweeping strokes from the waist to the shoulders. Then either take time to stroke her back firmly, doing whatever feels natural, or follow the sequence described below. As long as you relax and enjoy it, she will, too.

□ With thumbs in the center of the back and fingers out to the side, run your thumbs up the spine with gentle but firm pressure and take the thumbs out across the shoulders to finish. Repeat five times.

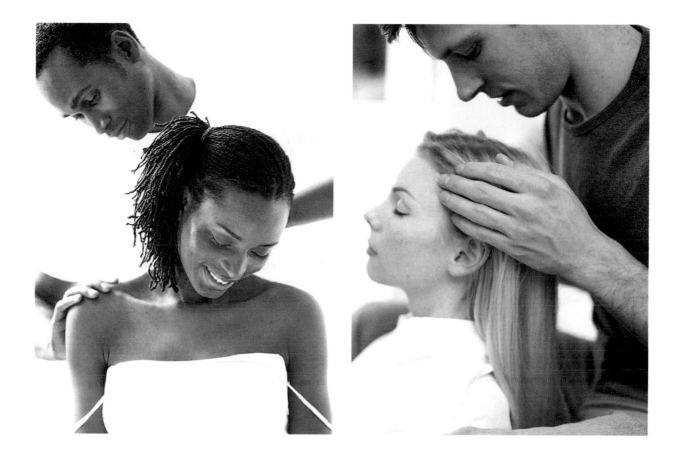

□ Sweep your hands over her back, applying pressure with the base of your palms. Repeat three times. Then repeat three times again, using tiny circular movements rather than a sweep of the hands, to ease away tension. Focus on the lower back and across the shoulders.

□ Place each thumb facing down on either side of her neck; slowly move them along the top of the shoulders; at the outer edge, press firmly. Repeat three times.

□ Finish by lightly pinching along the shoulders and gently gliding your hands over the entire back.

HAIR AND SCALP MASSAGE

When she is sitting comfortably, ask her to close her eyes and relax the neck and shoulders. Gently rub tiny circles along the shoulders and up the nape of the neck. Then, placing all your fingers in her hair, slowly massage the scalp; lift the hair up in your fingers and hold for a count of three. If her hair is short, pick up the hair between the fingers and close the fingers together so that she feel the hair being gently pulled. Repeat several times. The sensation is spine-tinglingly good.

rubbing the body when it **hurts** temporarily **wipes** away **pain** by blocking the **message** as it travels to the brain

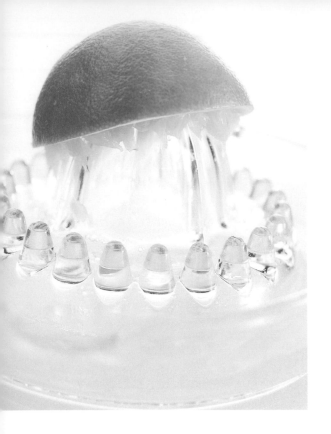

Never underestimate the importance of how you feel during these nine months. Seek out any mood-enhancing tips and tricks that make you feel good about *you*.

1 For just a few minutes every day, spend time communing with your baby. Baby meditation is an ancient tradition in China and Japan, where pregnant women would sit and meditate and communicate daily with their unborn babes, emphasizing the importance of the psychic and emotional link between mother and child. Breathe in deeply and let your limbs relax, then focus inwardly on your baby's presence. Slowly visualize his tiny body, the head, arms, legs, fingers, and toes. Try to imagine the warmth of the amniotic fluid, and the floating sensation that he must be experiencing.

TEN WAYS TO... *feel positive*

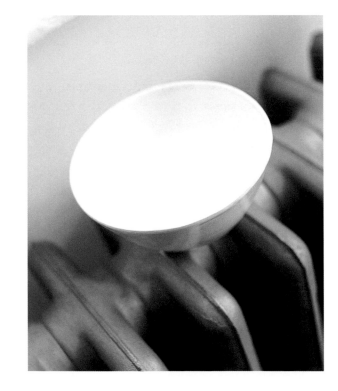

2 Visualization—the art of relaxation through positive mental imagery—is the most positive therapy imaginable. Breathe deeply, close your eyes, and focus your mind on a peaceful place you've been to—it could be a beach, a special tree from your childhood, your Dad's lap, or a hilltop—anywhere that's important to you. Then imagine yourself there again.

3 Don't lose it. It isn't just your body that goes soft in pregnancy; your brain is often affected, too. Refresh mind and body by breathing deeply whenever you have a moment. It sends freshly oxygenated blood throughout your body, and boosts mental clarity.

4 Just because the sun isn't shining, don't fall into the trap of staying wrapped up inside. Get as much fresh air as you can—take a drive in the country, and walk in peace, giving you time and space to think.

5 Don't reserve deep breathing for labor; you can use it to calm your whole body when you feel tense and under pressure. Sit upright in a comfortable chair, with your hands resting on your bump. Breathe in fully, count to two, then breathe out for a count of six at the same rate. Be aware of your hands rising and falling.

6 When your baby kicks at you, tap back twice. Now you have made a connection. Whenever it happens, try to remember to respond with a tap or a stroke. If you communicate before the birth, you are half way to being bonded before your baby's even arrived. It's your mothering instinct—so trust it.

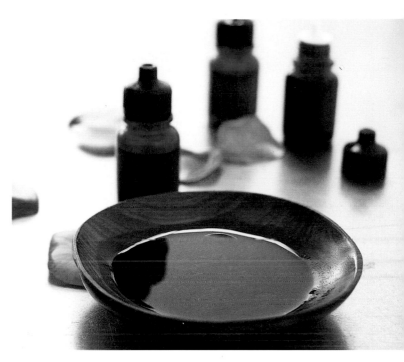

7 Enjoy the delights of rosewood essential oil. Bathe in it (5 drops), massage yourself with it (5 drops in 10 ml/2 tsp of carrier oil), inhale it, soothe your soul with a warm compress steeped in it (2 drops in a basin full of warm water), or burn it in a diffuser.

8 Immerse yourself in the color orange, which is energizing and believed by color therapists to help lift anxiety and depression. Eat several oranges, drink orange juice, wear the color either in clothing or perhaps as a piece of jewelry or woven twine as a wristband. Imagine sitting beneath an orange waterfall.

9 Add 2 drops of an essential oil of your choice to a large bowl of hand-hot water. Soak your hands or feet in the water for up to 15 minutes, and top up with warm water if it gets cool. Dry off with a towel and wrap up for another 15 minutes.

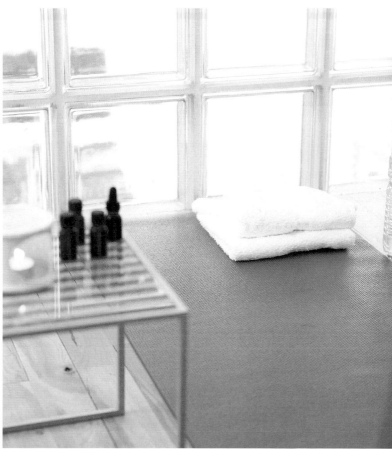

10 Close your eyes and place your left hand over the bridge of your nose, palm down, then stroke your palms outward, one over the other up your forehead and onto the hairline. Next take your fingertips into your scalp and using clawlike movements, massage your whole scalp. Repeat five times. Use a little face cream or oil to avoid dragging the skin.

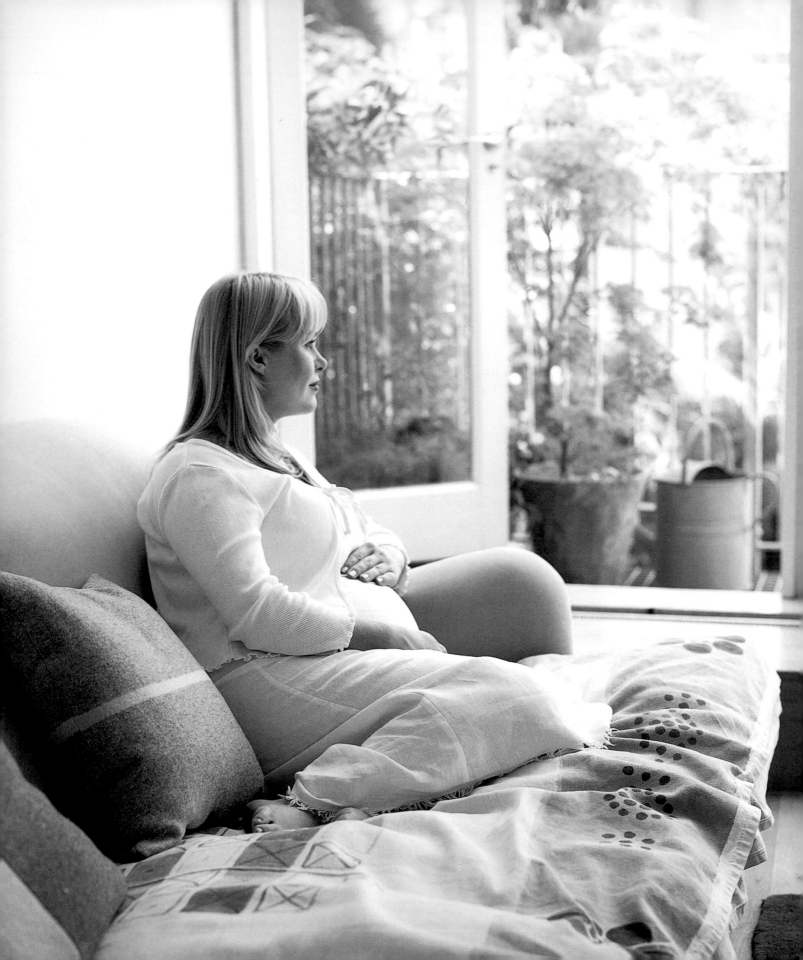

relax and prepare

Excitement and elation, fear and trepidation—you will experience the whole gamut of emotions in these last few weeks. Just remember that the best thing for your baby is that you should feel the best you can. Find effective ways to relax and unwind, to dwell and reflect on what's to come, and—above all—to enjoy. You are nearly there.

your changing body

Women carry their babies differently, and there are no rules about what is "normal." If this is a second or subsequent baby, you may appear bigger earlier in the pregnancy. Whatever your size, shape, or weight gain, remember that you and your evolving body are beautiful and blooming, and you should embrace and enjoy your new shape as much as possible.

DRESSING IN WINTER AND SUMMER

Dressing for a winter pregnancy is harder than you might imagine. For one thing, you won't feel the cold as much as everyone else. Then, of all the items of clothing to buy in pregnancy, a coat is the most expensive—so do you buy a "tent" for the third trimester? My advice is to wear a lightweight raincoat over loose-fitting, light layers, so you can vary how much you're wearing according to the temperature of the room you're in.

Depending on how much weight you have put on, dressing for a summer pregnancy is generally easier. If you need extra confidence to bare your flesh, use a fake tan to take the edge off pasty skin. It makes you look and feel brighter and healthier, and is considered to be safe in pregnancy.

SOOTHING YOUR SKIN

Itchy skin is common in pregnancy, especially on your bump, and this is not only because your skin is more sensitive, but also because bile salts are not metabolized well in pregnancy, especially after six months. There are several things you can do to help yourself.

□ Drink plenty of water to flush out your system.

□ Apply a cooling, soothing lotion such as calamine.

□ Half a cupful of bicarbonate of soda in a warm bath may help to soothe your skin.

□ Avoid using soap on your skin, which can be drying and make it more itchy. Try aqueous cream instead—the purest cleanser for your skin.

□ In your third trimester only, mix 3 drops of Roman chamomile with 1 drop of lavender in 10 ml (2 tsp) of almond oil. Keep in an airtight bottle and massage into the affected area whenever it gets itchy.

COLOSTRUM

You may find that from around six months you leak a little colostrum (the baby's first milk) from your nipples. It can be alarming if you don't know what it is, but this is simply your body preparing itself for the arrival of the baby. If it doesn't happen, there is no reason to worry.

"I remember wanting to wear a silk figure-hugging dress—but my belly button had just popped out. At the party one friend commented that my belly button was still flat. 'That's because I've taped it down,' I replied. Well, it worked, and I felt fabulous in my dress."

CORINNA, MOTHER OF KATIE AND CHARLOTTE

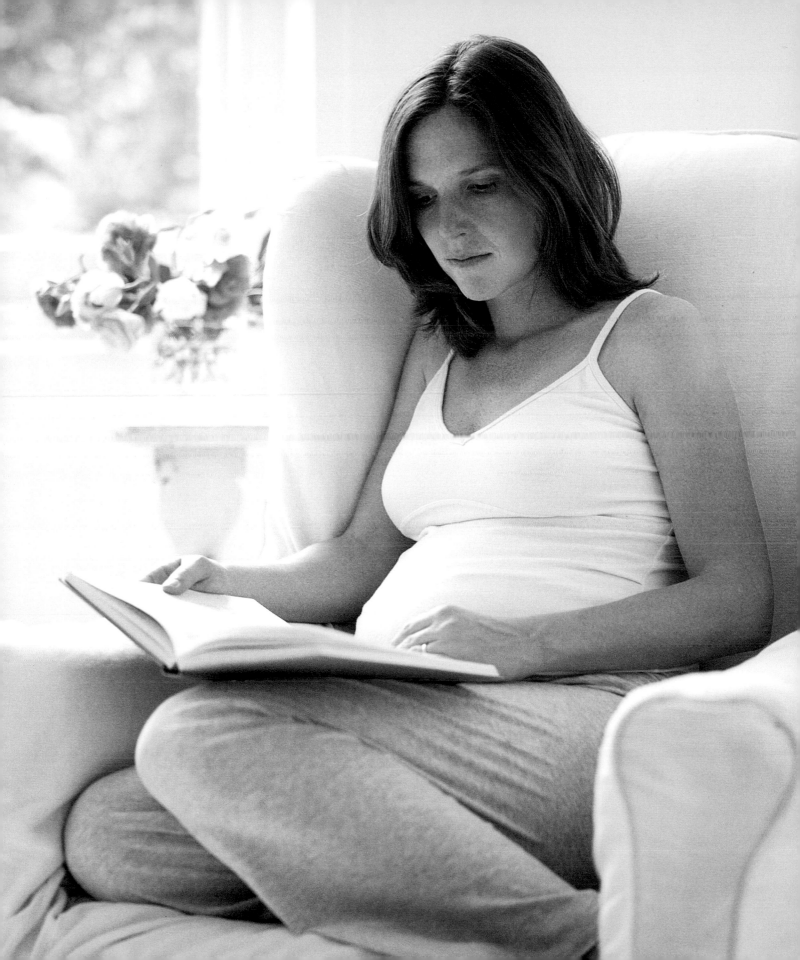

if you keep your **legs** looking great, you can wear **fashionable** and **attractive** styles all the **way** through your **pregnancy**

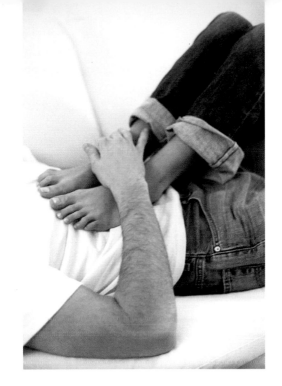

looking after your legs

In my opinion, "resting" during pregnancy is not really about nurturing the baby at all; it's about preserving the veins in your legs. Remember these words: "Don't stand when you can sit; don't sit when you can lie down"—and get yourself horizontal a bit more often.

IN GOOD SHAPE

Fit, firm, shapely legs prior to pregnancy can carry you stylishly through the whole nine months. If you eat a healthy, well-balanced diet in pregnancy, they shouldn't put on much more weight, staying pretty much the same size and shape as they were before conception. Great legs can also help you to wear certain styles that allow you to feel more attractive and fashionable all the way through. And for those of us who are less than blessed from the waist down, regular foot and leg exercises can help to keep your legs feeling lighter and more comfortable during a long day on your feet.

RESTLESS LEGS

Your legs ache and ache, and you don't know where to put them for comfort. One solution is to raise them often. Another is to stimulate them by massage. Using firm strokes, massage in a little lotion, cream, or oil. Start from your soles, applying gentle pressure to the arches and between the toes. Gently stroke your legs upward from the ankle to the knee, finishing with firm pressure behind the knee. An energizing leg cream with menthol might help to cool and relax your legs, too.

EDEMA

Swelling of the legs and ankles, called edema, is caused by an increase in fluid retention in the body, especially in the lower limbs. This is due to the pressure of the uterus on the vessels that return blood from the lower parts of the body to the heart. You may notice that your shoes feel tight and the skin looks and feels stretched, especially at the end of the day or in hot weather, and it can become really uncomfortable. Any swelling should always be monitored carefully since, when accompanied by high blood pressure and protein in the urine, it may be a symptom of pre-eclampsia.

□ Avoid standing for long periods of time and, whenever you can, rest on your bed for an hour with your feet raised to a level higher than your heart.

□ It may help to wear maternity support pantyhose. Avoid wearing hold-ups or tight socks or shoes that dig into your skin.

□ Exercise can help to prevent swelling by improving the body's circulation. Try some gentle foot exercises: sit comfortably upright on a chair, stretch one foot out and gently rotate your ankle and foot to boost circulation. Repeat with the other foot.

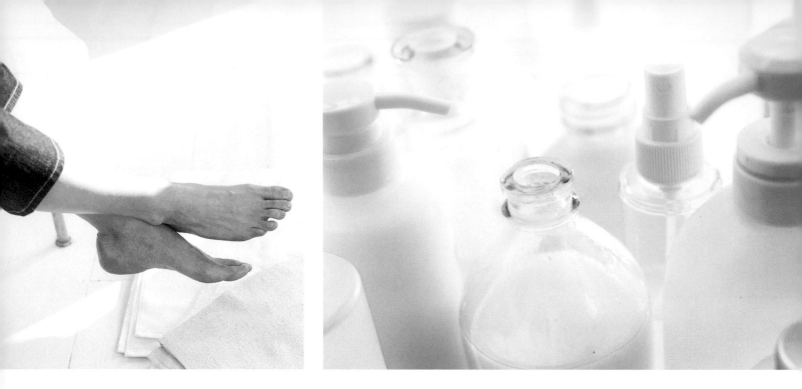

VARICOSE VEINS

Varicose veins are caused by increased venous pressure from carrying extra weight and by pregnancy hormones that soften blood vessel walls. If your mother had varicose veins, you may be predisposed to get them. To help to prevent them, take the following measures.

□ Exercise regularly.

□ Avoid standing for long periods.

□ Cross your legs at the ankles, not at the knees.

□ Try to avoid gaining too much weight.

□ Avoid wearing anything tight or constricting.

CRAMP

Cramp is common in pregnancy. Causes include circulatory changes and lack of calcium—or it may simply be caused by increased pressure from extra weight on the leg muscles and circulatory system. There are several effective ways to alleviate cramp.

□ Try this shiatsu technique to bring relief from cramp and prevent further episodes. Flex your foot. Locate the liver point 4 (LIV4) on the inside of the foot, in the area between the tendon and the anklebone. Press the point for 5 to 10 seconds, then relax. Repeat three times.

□ As the cramp occurs, slowly sip this homeopathic remedy: four tablets of Magnesia phosphorica 6C dissolved in a glass of warm water.

□ Instead of pointing your toes to relieve the pain, pull your foot back toward you.

□ To treat frequent episodes of cramp, try acupuncture or osteopathy.

□ Exercise regularly.

□ Try calcium and magnesium supplements.

give your legs a **stimulating** massage: using **firm** strokes, massage in a little **lotion**, cream, or oil—start from the **soles** of your feet, applying **gentle** pressure

CELLULITE

Cellulite hits hardest during puberty and pregnancy, thanks to those delightful feminine hormones. Pregnancy is not the time to diet, but a healthy eating plan that features more fresh fruit and vegetables and fewer sugary snacks will not only give you more energy during pregnancy, but may also help to reduce the amount of cellulite you develop. Save dieting for later.

COSMETIC CARE

When you simply can't reach any more and waxing isn't an option, get your partner to shave your legs for you.

This may sound unappealing on first consideration, but if you set the mood and tell him how sympathetic and wonderful he is, you will soon discover that he is pretty good at it.

Clipping toenails is almost impossible once you are in the last trimester, and it becomes all too easy for your poor feet to get neglected. Ask another favor from your partner—or treat yourself to a professional pedicure. It's a small price to pay for making you and your toes feel prettier and more comfortable. Your feet have more nerve endings than any other part of your body, so they will respond well to a bit of pampering.

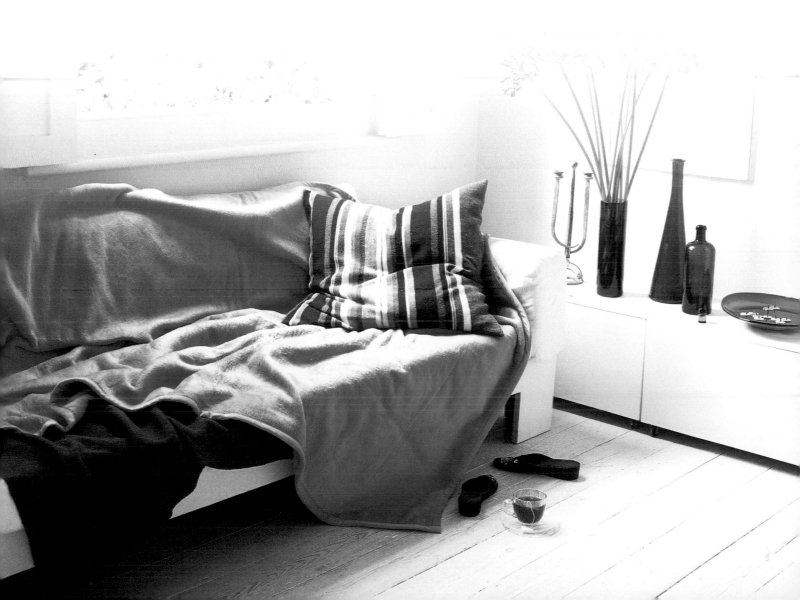

keeping up the body work

You have reached the home stretch, with just the last few weeks to go, but you may be getting less sleep than you did earlier in the pregnancy and be feeling devoid of energy. If that is the case, there are plenty of ways to keep yourself looking and feeling your very best right up to the delivery day.

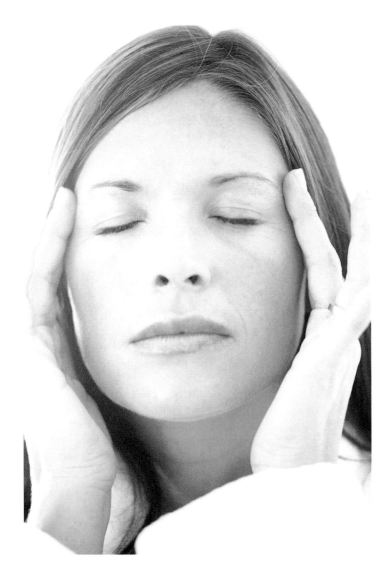

OPENING YOUR EYES

The visible consequence of poor-quality sleep—tired, puffy eyes or dark circles—is enough to make look as if you've been up all night. Sorry—that is meant to be after you've had your dear little bundle, isn't it? A little morning puffiness and fluid retention that has built up over the third trimester not only affects your body, but can also make your eyes feel more sensitive.

Increased fluid levels in pregnancy frequently cause water retention, making the eyes swell so they appear puffier than usual. This may also mean a change of prescription for wearers of glasses or contact lenses. An increase in hormones leads to more protein deposits in the tears, which makes wearing contact lenses less comfortable, too.

Get an eye test. Your eyes may not only become irritated and contact lenses less comfortable to wear, but your eyes may become more farsighted, which will obviously affect your prescription.

Optometrists recommend wearing glasses or opting for the more hygienic disposable or daily-wear lenses for comfort and eye health. If it is a problem for you, reduce the amount of time you wear contact lenses during pregnancy.

□ If puffy eyes are a problem, try using an extra pillow to raise your head in bed, and try to sleep on your back to help prevent fluid from "pooling" around the eyes.

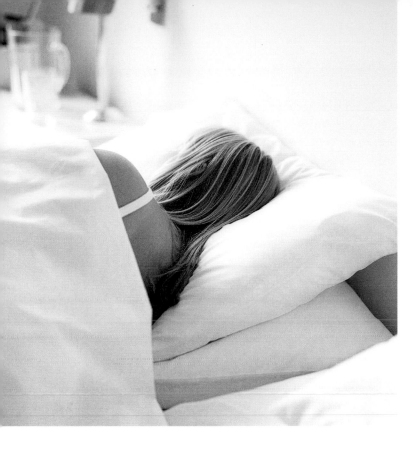

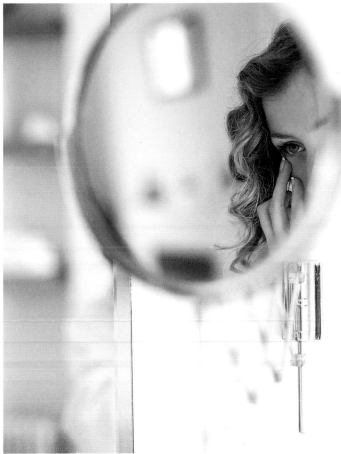

□ Try "palming," a gentle massage to stop puffiness. With fingers pointing up toward the top of your head, gently press the heels of your hands onto the tops of the cheekbones. Rest the palms gently on the eyelids so you can feel the heat they generate.

□ Cover up dark circles with a light-reflective concealer. Hold a mirror in front of you, and, keeping your chin lowered, look up into it so you can see clearly where your dark circles need concealing. Pat concealer onto the dark areas only, then blend lightly with your finger.

□ Curl your eyelashes—believe it or not, it really can help to make your eyes look more wide-awake. Curling the lashes upwards "opens up" the eye. Straight lashes that look downward only make you look sleepier.

□ Get moving. Activity improves circulation and in turn improves puffiness and dark circles.

"I found that the one item of makeup I really couldn't do without during pregnancy was my concealer. It helped to hide how little sleep I'd had."

RACHEL, MOTHER OF EVIE AND JOSHUA

NURTURING YOUR SKIN

When your skin has been looking its best for months, it is easy to forget that all those hormones are about to revert back to their previous levels. Establish a skincare regime, now, that you can sustain after the birth.

□ Continue to apply a sunblock before going in the sun to protect your skin fully and minimize melasma (see page 19). Choose an SPF 25+ in cloudy or clear skies.

□ Treat yourself to a skin-nurturing facial. Remind the therapist that you are pregnant—especially if she is using any essential oils. Or try giving yourself a facial at home (see Rose Facial Massage, right).

□ Book a professional massage. You should be relaxing and pampering both yourself and baby right now, and all that oil is great for your skin. As you get bigger, you may worry that a massage could be uncomfortable, but you can be massaged straddled across a chair or lying on your side or on a beanbag—whatever you prefer.

□ Practice deep breathing for healthier-looking skin. Lie back against cushions, with your knees raised on a pillow or cushion. Breathe in and out slowly and evenly from the tummy, not the chest; with each breath out, sigh and try to relax and empty your mind. Do this for five to ten minutes. At no point should you feel faint or dizzy. If you do, stop and resume your usual breathing pattern until the faintness or dizziness has subsided.

ROSE FACIAL MASSAGE

The best time to massage your face is while applying nourishing face oil. Mix 1 drop of rose essential oil with 5 ml (1 tsp) of almond or wheatgerm oil and massage gently into your face, keeping away from the eyes.

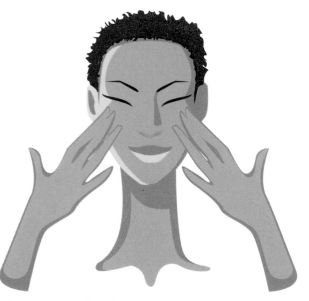

TO BRIGHTEN YOUR SKIN

Starting at the brows, massage each part of your face, using tiny sweeping upward movements. There are five steps: from brows to temples, forehead to hairline, eyes to ears, sides of the nose to the ears (above), and chin to ears (right).

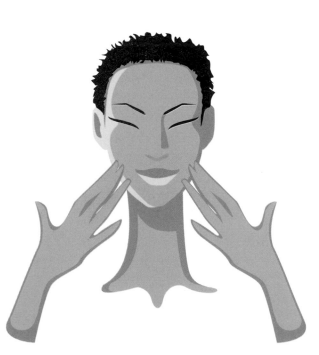

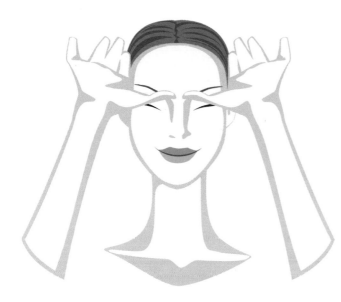

TO SMOOTH YOUR FOREHEAD

Stroke the bridge of your nose with upward sweeps of your thumbs (left). Switch to your first two fingers and press and stroke over the entire brow from inner to outer edges (below). Finish off on the temples—press twice, and relax.

TO BRIGHTEN YOUR EYES

Press at small, regular intervals from the inner corners of the eyes, beneath the eyes and out over the cheeks to the temples (left). Repeat twice, pressing lower and lower each time, until you press under the cheekbones for the final time.

establish a **skincare** regime now that will keep you looking **glowing** and **radiant** even after the birth, when **your** hormone levels start to revert to **normal**

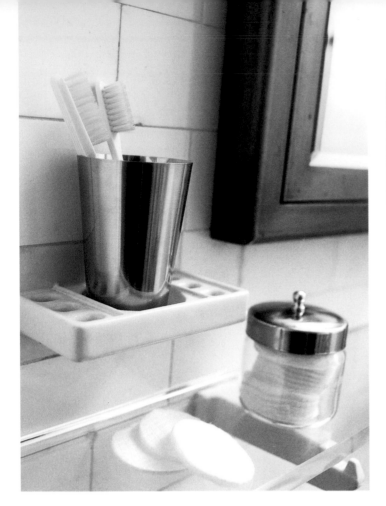

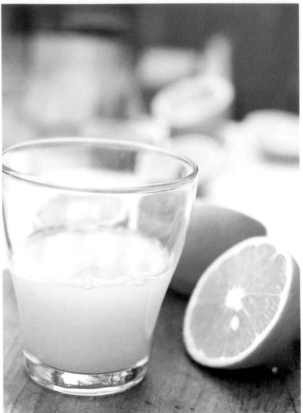

LOOKING AFTER YOUR TEETH

There are many myths about what happens to women's teeth in pregnancy. In the past, less was known about gingivitis, or gum disease, and when a pregnant woman lost a tooth, the baby was blamed for depriving her of calcium; we now know that a baby does not deplete its mother of enough calcium to affect her teeth. It is the increase in blood supply in a woman's body during pregnancy that causes gums to swell and become soft and spongy, so they tend to bleed more easily. Pregnancy also makes you more sensitive to plaque.

Studies have demonstrated that pregnant women with severe gingivitis at the time of delivery were more than twice as likely to develop pre-eclampsia than those with healthy gums. The theory is that gum disease may cause an infection in the bloodstream. So take extra care of your teeth at this time.

☐ Floss regularly to remove plaque and visit a hygienist once in each trimester; dental tape is softer than floss.
☐ If your gums bleed when you brush your teeth, rinse your mouth with a solution of warm water and sea salt.
☐ Try rubbing a small amount of the homeopathic tincture Hypercal (a herbal mixture of hypericum and calendula) into the affected areas.
☐ Eat plenty of foods rich in vitamin C, such as citrus fruits, strawberries, kiwi fruits, broccoli, cabbage, and potatoes, and take a vitamin C supplement.
☐ Avoid sugary or overprocessed foods and soft drinks that encourage plaque.
☐ You may be concerned about the safety of X-rays, but in dentistry the beam is so small and accurate that it just goes in the cheek and out the other side. Consult your dentist before having an X-ray, and consider leaving any major dental treatment until after the birth.

STAYING COMFORTABLE

Many women find that they expand beyond their expectations in the third trimester. The weight of the baby places an even greater strain on various veins and nerves (most commonly, the sciatic nerve in the legs), making you feel heavy and uncomfortable at times throughout the day, and may cause some additional minor discomfort. Your abdominal area may also feel quite sensitive because muscles and ligaments are being stretched to their limit.

Common problems at this stage of pregnancy include excessive itchiness across the abdomen and a rash between the thighs caused by heat and friction.
□ Wear loose, comfortable slacks to prevent your legs from rubbing together. It may keep you cooler, too.
□ Frequent showers will keep you cool and fresh, but avoid using soap on sensitive rashes.
□ Apply a soothing cream such as chamomile ointment (better known for its usefulness after the birth than before), which is a fabulous cream for minor rashes and skin irritations, and is especially effective for treating diaper rash.

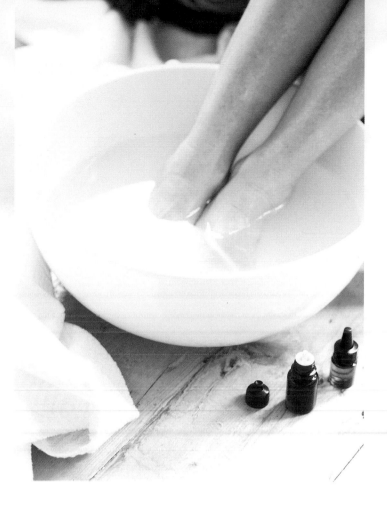

SUPPORTING YOUR BREASTS

Breasts may develop occasional rashes and skin tags. Although some rashes may be due to a raised body temperature and hot weather, others have no obvious cause. Skin changes are inevitable at this time because of the increased level of hormones flooding through your body. Women with heavier breasts may prefer to wear a lightweight bra in bed for extra support (remember, no underwire). Condition the skin well, too, since breasts in pregnancy and while breastfeeding are as susceptible to stretch marks as the abdominal area.
□ Wash your breasts at least twice daily to keep your skin cool and fresh, especially on the underside of your breasts.
□ A bra with good support will help to prevent back pain and minimize stretch marks. A sports bra is a wonderful alternative to a maternity bra, especially for women with larger breasts.

do **everything** you can to keep your body **feeling** fresh and **light** from **top** to toe—cool down quickly by **immersing** your **feet** in a bowl of **cool water**

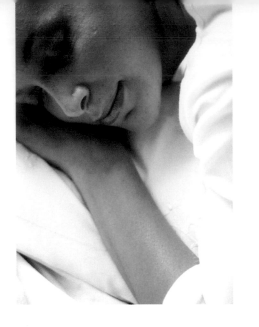

One odd thing about being pregnant is that you always seem to feel hotter than everyone else around you, whether it's summer or winter. Here are some invaluable ways to keep your cool, at home or at work, so you feel comfortable and in control of your pregnancy.

TEN WAYS TO...*stay cool*

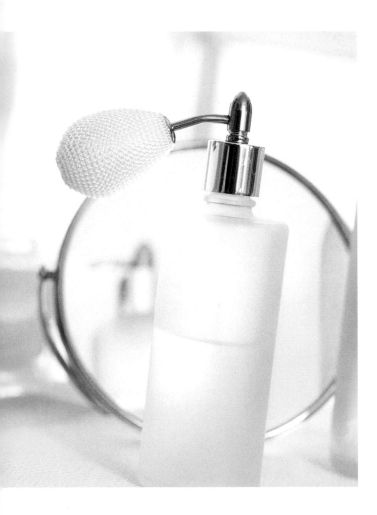

1 Wear loose, floaty clothing (preferably dresses) that won't constrict you around the middle as you expand further.

2 An icy-cold damp cloth on the nape of the neck brings down your entire body temperature—or try running cold water over your wrists to cool your body.

3 If you don't have air conditioning in your home, either open your refrigerator door for a quick cool-down (à la Marilyn Monroe) or, better still, go to the supermarket and loiter by the open freezer compartments whenever you get the chance.

4 Keep your skin care in the fridge. This may sound crazy, but if your eye cream, cleanser, toner, and moisturizer are really cool first thing, it's a more positive way to start the day, and it instantly perks up the skin.

5 Sip several cups of peppermint tea throughout the day. It is cooling to the body and helps soothe digestion. Look for a peppermint foot lotion, which immediately helps to cool the skin.

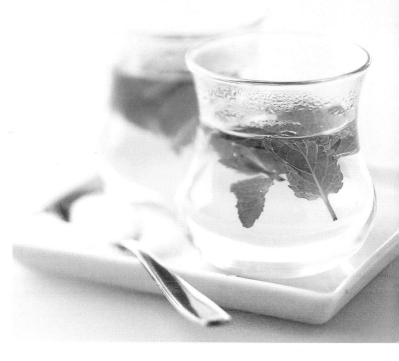

6 If you need to wear hose at your place of work, make sure that they don't constrict you too much, and apply a cooling leg gel under or through the pantyhose during the day to relieve that sensation of "restless legs." If you work all day in an office, raise up your feet under your desk to help prevent puffiness, but don't raise them higher than the bump.

7 Avoid going out in the sun around midday—you may underestimate just how hot it is, and it could make you feel dizzy and nauseous. And don't sunbathe your baby on vacation. Experts say that you are hotter than usual when pregnant, and intense heat may actually cause the fetus to get a fever. Avoid tanning salons during pregnancy. The heat from the concentrated ultraviolet rays—let alone the radiation itself—may be damaging to the fetus.

8 Carry a facial spray around with you when you're traveling in the car or on public transportation. Buy an empty spray bottle and fill with mineral water or rosewater, or just add a few favorite essential oils such as 2 drops each of lavender and chamomile to a bottle of mineral water and spritz throughout the day. It smells divine and doubles up as a natural fragrance when your nose gets too sensitive to the one you usually wear.

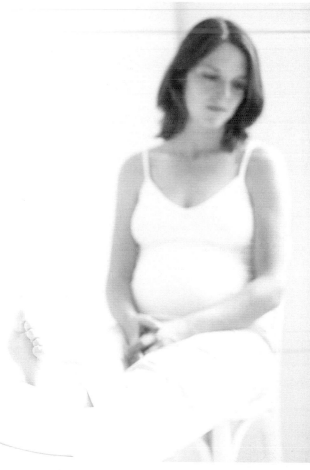

9 When you get home at the end of a hot day, or if the heat is just too intense to bear, plunge your feet straight into a bowl of cool water. Do this as often as you need.

10 Change the way you sleep to help you keep your cool. Open the windows an hour before you go to bed. A well-ventilated room will help you sleep better. Sleep between crisp clean cotton or linen sheets that are cooler than manmade alternatives. And invest in an efficient fan—you may find that it is impossible to sleep without one.

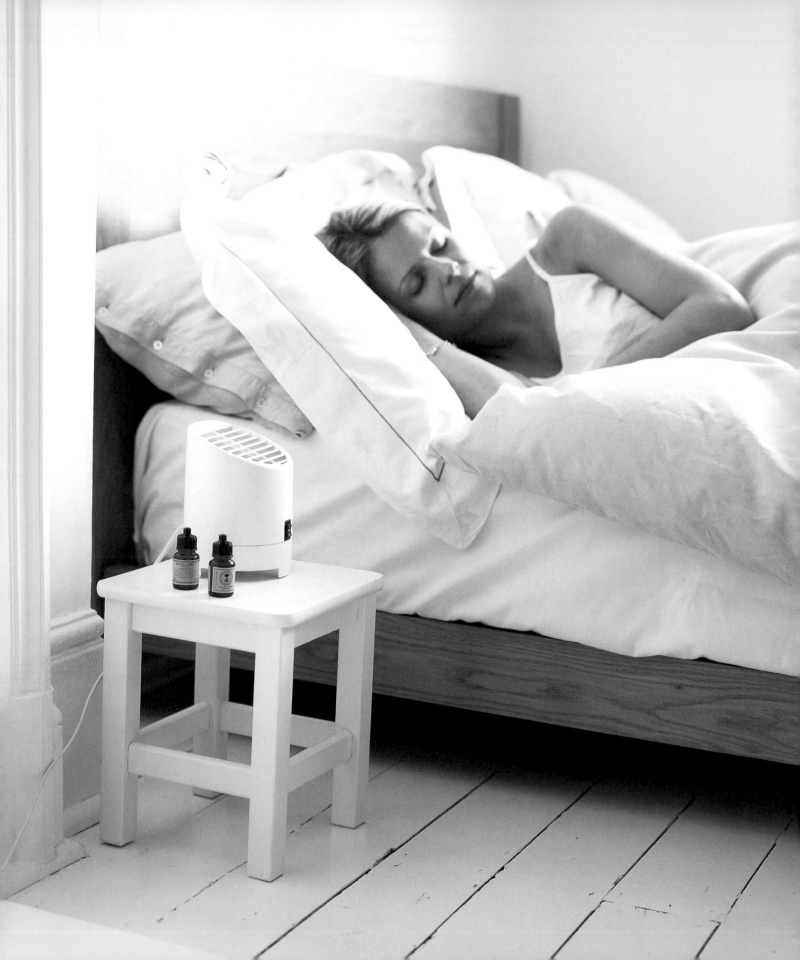

getting a good night's sleep

In the last trimester it's hard enough to sleep at night because you just can't seem to get comfortable, let alone the fact that "someone else" thinks it's time to wake up and play footsie with your bladder and kidneys. And if the weather is hot—forget it. But there are plenty of things you can do to make sleep come more easily.

DEEP-SLEEP STRATEGY

The most effective way to get yourself in the mood for sleep is to indulge in a relaxing bedtime ritual. This could incorporate some or all of the following elements.

□ Put 3 drops of frankincense, sandalwood, or neroli oil in a vaporizer in your bedroom before going to bed.

□ Play a relaxation tape or a relaxing piece of music.

□ Arrange pillows and cushions so that you are in the most comfortable position (one behind your back and one under bent knees helps to support your back).

□ Massage your tummy with the wonderful aromatic Balance Blend (see page 61).

□ Try this relaxation technique. Close your eyes and take a deep breath. Keep breathing slowly, aware of the rhythm. Focus on each part of your body, starting with the right foot, breathing into any tension and releasing it. Work up the right leg. Then focus on your left side, followed by your bottom, hips, and each section of your back. Breathe into and relax your tummy and chest. Relax your right hand up the arm to the shoulder, then your left hand up the arm to the shoulder. Breathe slowly and deeply. Relax your neck and release tension from the jaw, cheeks, temples, forehead, and the back of the head up to the crown. Take a long deep breath. Note how your body feels heavy and totally relaxed. Focus again on the rhythm of your breathing. Stay like this for as long as is comfortable. When you are ready, start moving your fingers and toes and stretch out as you breathe deeply.

COMFORT TIPS FOR SLEEPING OR RELAXATION

One of the most important conditions for peaceful sleep and relaxation is comfort.

□ Lie on your side with a pillow between your knees to reduce the strain on your ligaments. You may want to put another pillow under your bump, too.

□ Prop yourself up on two or three pillows or on a beanbag to relieve any strain on your lower back. This position is also good for relieving heartburn.

□ Sit in an armchair with a V-shaped pillow supporting your head. Use a small stool to support your lower legs. Put a pillow on the stool for extra comfort.

□ Keep a bottle of water by your bed; dehydration at night can cause headaches by morning.

focus on the **rhythm** of your breathing as you **release** the **tension** from your body

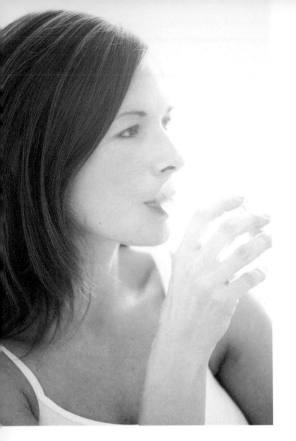

"From 36 weeks of my third pregnancy, I spent two weeks in bed doubled up in agony, and was in and out of hospital with a suspected early onset of labor. Finally a friend asked if I might be constipated. I was in so much pain I never dreamt that was the cause. But it was."

JO, MOTHER OF KATHERINE AND ELSA

coping with ailments

There are a variety of minor ailments that occur in pregnancy which —even though they do no harm to you or your baby—can be incredibly uncomfortable and difficult to bear at times. Just remember that heartburn, constipation, and similar afflictions are extremely common and won't last.

HEARTBURN

Heartburn, or indigestion, is a burning pain in your chest or a sour taste in your mouth caused by acid from partly digested food "burning" your esophagus.

how you can help yourself

□ Avoid spicy and fatty foods, and eat little and often.

□ Drink separately from eating so that your stomach does not get too full.

□ At the first sign of heartburn, have an alkaline drink, such as milk, to neutralize the acid effect (but note that milk may cause heartburn in some people). Antacid preparations can help, but consult your doctor first.

□ Relax after eating. Avoid exercising or bending over for about 30 minutes to an hour after a meal, until your food has been sufficiently digested.

CONSTIPATION

Constipation is surprisingly uncomfortable and becomes increasing common as pregnancy progresses, due to hormonal changes that now cause food and waste to pass more slowly than before through your digestive system. If you have been prescribed iron supplements for anemia at around this time, they will exacerbate the condition.

how you can help yourself

□ Increase your intake of fiber (drinking prune juice is natural and effective).

□ Consider how you can reduce your stress levels. An aromatherapy massage using neroli oil on the belly, in a clockwise direction (following the path of the large intestine), is good for calming and destressing.

□ Reduce your intake of dairy and wheat products, which clog up the intestines. Eat plenty of fresh fruit and vegetables, chew your food slowly, and drink plenty of mineral water and fruit teas between meals.

□ Acupuncture and shiatsu are both good at releasing blocked energy in the body.

□ Homeopaths recommend taking Nux Vomica 6C three times a day for a week.

HEMORRHOIDS

Hemorrhoids (or piles) are common in late pregnancy and can cause much discomfort. They are swollen veins in the rectum or around the anus caused by extra pressure; they may be itchy and painful or may bleed.

how you can help yourself

□ For fast relief, an over-the-counter cream applied topically will work within a few days.

□ Avoid straining on the toilet.

□ Drink plenty of fluids to avoid constipation and the need to strain.

□ Warm baths are soothing, but avoid hot baths, which make the blood vessels dilate.

□ Increase your intake of vitamins C, E, and B6 as a preventive measure.

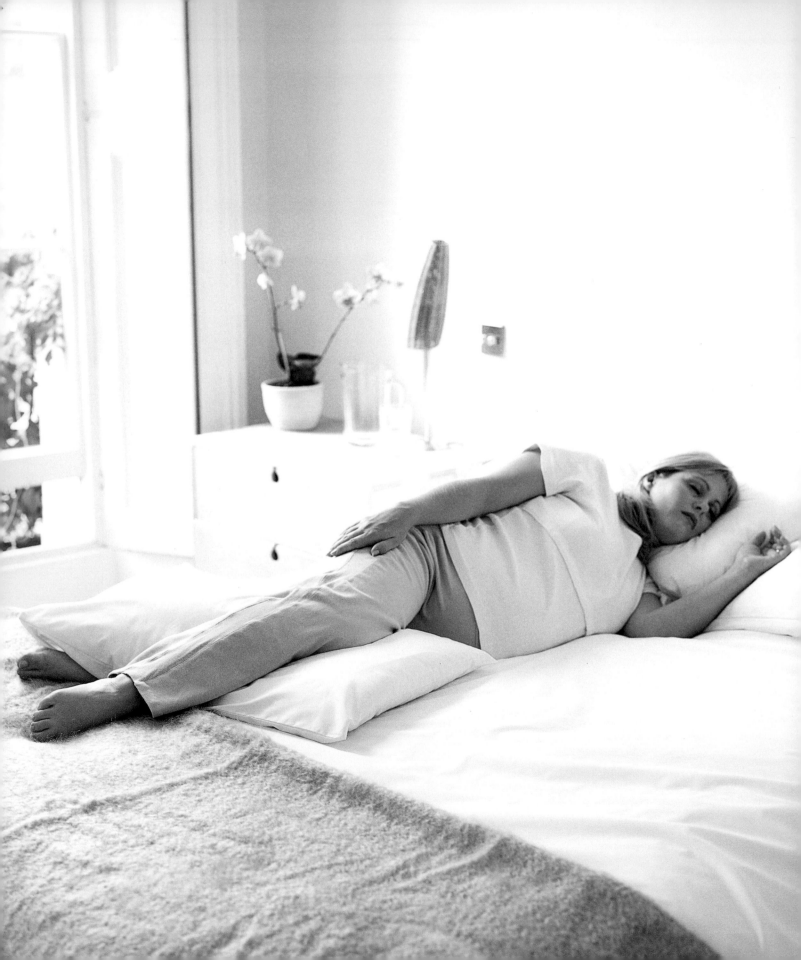

FAINTING

Fainting or feeling light-headed and dizzy is usually caused by low blood pressure or low blood sugar levels. If it occurs more than once or twice in your pregnancy, seek medical advice from your doctor.

how you can help yourself

□ If you feel faint, try lying on your side with a pillow tucked between your knees and breathe deeply.

□ Inhale a reviving, energizing aroma such as orange, mandarin, or grapefruit.

□ To prevent dizziness, try the soldier's trick: stand up and press down on the balls of your feet.

□ Keep a healthy snack such as a banana on hand to help maintain blood sugar levels between meals.

STRESS INCONTINENCE

Stress incontinence may occur during the late months of pregnancy if this is your first baby—and at any time during the nine months if you have already had a baby. It is caused by the extra weight and pressure on the bladder from the baby, combined with weakened pelvic floor muscles, causing you to "leak" some urine when you cough, sneeze, or laugh.

how you can help yourself

□ Make sure that you do your pelvic-floor exercises (see page 68).

□ Don't try to "hold on" if your bladder is full.

□ If you feel the urge to empty your bladder even though you have just done so, practice your pelvic-floor exercises. Stress incontinence will improve, but only with exercise.

□ If you continue to have trouble after birth—when stress incontinence is often more pronounced—ask your doctor for a referral to a urologist.

BLADDER INFECTIONS

It is common to feel the need to urinate more often at the beginning and end of pregnancy, but if you feel discomfort while doing so, you may have a bladder infection (cystitis) or a kidney infection (pyelitis), which causes pain around the lower back and kidney area. Seek medical advice if you think you have an infection.

how you can help yourself

□ Keep up your fluid intake at all times. Drink a glass of water every time you go to the toilet, even at night.

□ Cranberry juice and grapefruit juice are believed to help prevent bladder infections—or try drinking marshmallow tea.

□ Try to empty your bladder as much as you can every time you go to the toilet.

OOH!

At any time in the third trimester, you may feel a tense tightening across your bump, which feels rigid and firm to the touch for about 30 seconds. This is a Braxton-Hicks contraction, which is like a practice contraction, toning up the uterus ready for birth. Some women barely notice Braxton-Hicks contractions; in others (especially those who have already had a child), they are more pronounced. If you feel pain at the same time, check with your doctor or midwife to make sure you are not going into premature labor.

the first time you experience a **Braxton-Hicks**—a tense **tightening** across your bump—you could be forgiven **for thinking** that you are in labor

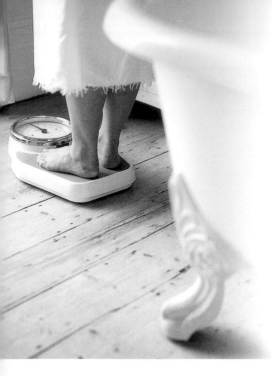

gaining weight: how much?

Naturally, it is important that you put on weight while you are pregnant. Part of the weight gain is caused by the laying down of fat in preparation for milk production and breastfeeding. Some women may pile on weight in the first trimester while trying to stave off nausea from morning sickness; others may find they lose weight at this stage—and put it on later; others simply put on weight steadily throughout the pregnancy. We are all individual.

LISTEN TO YOUR BODY

What you must not do is to go against what your body tells you. If your body says rest, you must rest. If your body says eat, you must eat. This is not the time for slimming. If you eat a well-balanced diet that is not too high in sugary, fatty foods, you will put on the right amount of weight for your height and shape.

Most women will have gained something between 22 and 33 lb (10 and 15 kg) by the end of the nine months. This weight takes into account the weight of the baby at birth, the placenta, the fluids around the baby, and vital fat stores. If you put on a bit more,

it will simply be harder to lose, but there is no point in admonishing yourself over a few cookies. But some women who put on too much weight develop gestational diabetes (pregnancy diabetes, which increases the risk of diabetes later in life), and in such a case the baby risks becoming diabetic, too. If prenatal tests show that you are at risk of developing gestational diabetes, you may have to have further tests and be put on a special diet to control your blood sugar.

Stay in tune with your body. If you are eating well, you will feel well. If you are eating junk, you will feel tired, sluggish, and emotional.

YOUR TOTAL MINIMUM WEIGHT GAIN IN PREGNANCY

For a baby weighing 7.5 lb (3.4 kg) or 9 lb (4.1 kg) at birth—this is how the mother's estimated total weight gain in pregnancy of 20 lbs (9 kg) or 24 lb (10.8 kg) breaks down.

baby weight:		7.5 lb	9 lb
baby	38%	7.5 lb	9 lb
placenta	9%	1.8 lb	2.2 lb
amniotic fluid	12%	2.4 lb	2.9 lb
increased weight of breasts & uterus	19%	3.8 lb	4.4 lb
increased volume of blood	22%	4.4 1b	5.3 lb
estimated total weight gain		12.4 lb	23.8 lb

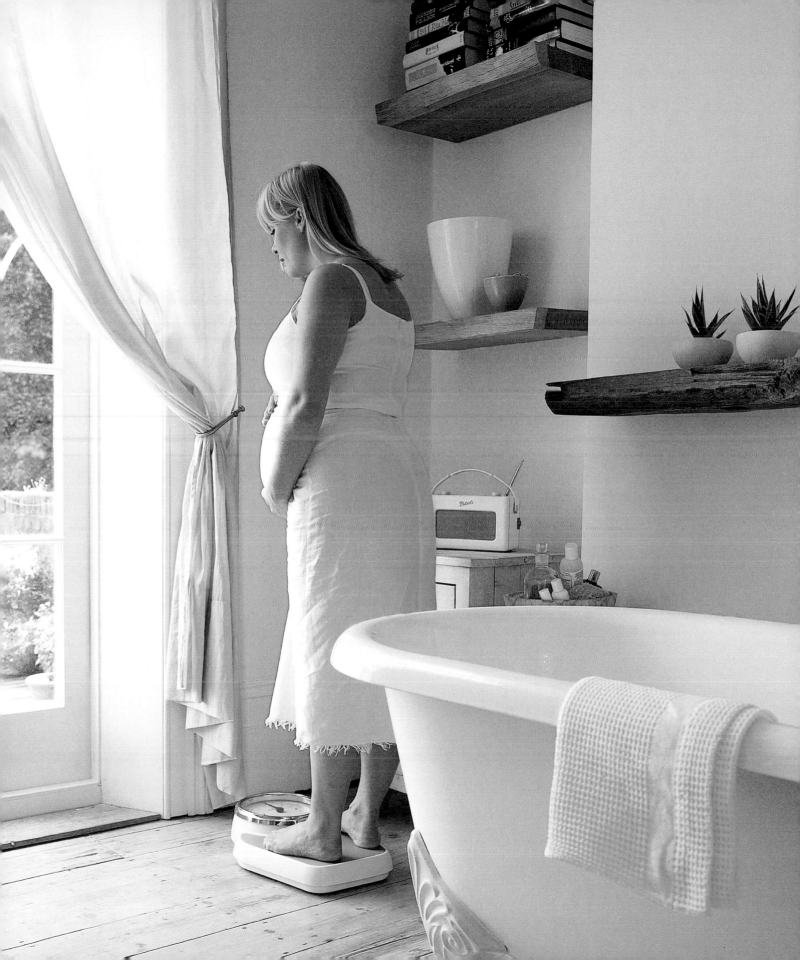

> "I carried on doing yoga throughout my second pregnancy and felt far fitter and better able to cope with the birth than I ever did with my first."
>
> **HELEN, MOTHER OF ELEANOR AND JACK**

enhancing the three Ss

These gentle pregnancy exercises are designed to keep you in tune with your body and enhance your strength, stamina, and suppleness in preparation for labor. But don't overextend yourself. Hormone-softened ligaments can easily be strained, so take everything nice and easy.

PREPARING TO STRETCH YOURSELF

Take advantage of a quiet time to expand your mind as you stretch your limbs. The benefits of gentle stretching go far beyond its effect on the body. Keep the room warm, empty your mind of daily worries and stressful thoughts, and focus on the positive: you and your baby. Use the floor, or a mat, if possible; play music if you prefer—and use this time for you. Try each exercise or just a couple, whatever suits you. You may find a great position to help you deal with labor pains, too.

FULL SQUAT

Keeping your back straight and legs apart, gradually squat down as low as is comfortable. Distribute your weight evenly between your heels and toes. Hold onto the back of a chair for support. Repeat 3 to 5 times.

PELVIC ROCK

Stand with your feet apart and knees slightly bent. Tighten your buttock muscles and tuck your "tail" under. Release your buttocks, then rock your pelvis backwards, keeping your upper body upright and knees bent. Now rock back and forth in this position, and side to side if comfortable. You may find this position is helpful at relieving backache when you are in labor.

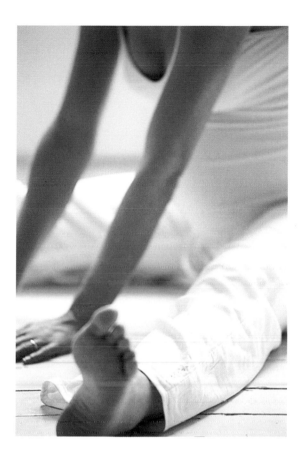

HALF-SQUAT

Hold onto a chair and place your right foot in front of your left (see left). Point your right knee slightly out and slowly bend both knees. Keep your bottom tucked in and your back straight. Stand up slowly. Repeat with the other leg in front. Repeat 3 to 5 times.

TUMMY TUCK

Lie flat on the floor, feet together and knees slightly bent (see below). Place a hand under the hollow of your back. Using your tummy muscles, press your spine against the floor until your back is flat, then slide your feet along the floor while keeping your back "glued" to the floor. When your back begins to arch, stop and relax with your knees bent again. Repeat 3 to 5 times.

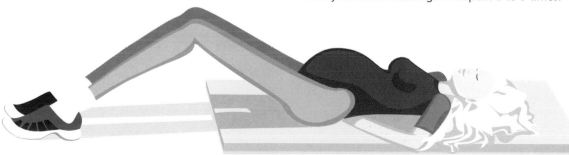

achieving a sense of calm

Worry and tiredness in the last months of pregnancy can bring on physical aches and pains as well as mental tension. This is the moment to concentrate on keeping calm.

ANXIETY

Anxiety—stirred up by fears about the birth, going into the hospital, or the baby's health—is normal. It can take the form of headaches, muscle aches and pains, tummy pains, panic attacks, and insomnia. Cranial osteopath is very calming and may help you to refocus, while acupuncture can help to rebalance your energy.

how you can help yourself

□ Bach Flower Rescue Remedy is excellent for relieving panic and tension.

□ Talk about any worries with your partner.

□ Yoga, deep breathing, meditation, and visualization can all help to alleviate tension and angst.

□ Aconite 30C homeopathic remedy is good for conquering fears. Take as directed.

□ Have a relaxing, warm bath containing 3 drops each of Roman chamomile and neroli essential oils.

INSOMNIA

Insomnia in pregnancy is often put down to discomfort, but it may also be linked to anxiety, indigestion, and overstimulation. Prolonged periods of disturbed sleep take their toll, and you should do what you can to get as much rest before the labor and birth, when you will need all the energy that you can muster.

how you can help yourself

□ Have a relaxing bath containing 2 drops each of Roman chamomile and tangerine essential oils.

□ A few drops of Bach Flower Rescue Remedy in a glass of water or on the tongue will calm you down.

□ Ask your partner to massage you with a relaxing aromatherapy oil such as the Relax Blend (page 61).

□ Drink a relaxing cup of chamomile tea before you go to bed at night, and try to avoid drinking tea and coffee throughout the day.

WATER THERAPY

When you are pregnant, water is one of the best natural soothers for both mind and body, and you may find it useful in labor, too. "Women in labor really relax in water," says Nicky Wales, senior midwife at the Active Birth Centre for Queen Charlotte's & Chelsea Hospital in London. "It's as good as gas and air. Doctors and nurses getting in the way of birth cause a lot of unnecessary intervention. Women push well in the pool and it keeps us away; leaving nature to get on with it."

FLORAL RELAXATION

For a great floral bath blend, add 3 drops of mandarin and 2 drops of neroli oils to the water. Both are good for the skin and may help to prevent stretch marks. Sprinkle the essential oils onto the water's surface, then mix well just before getting in. Soak yourself for 15 minutes and do not use soap because it spoils the composition of the oils—and the benefits to you.

BATH-TIME TIPS

Take care not to expose your baby or yourself to risks in the bathroom.

□ Make sure the bath water is comfortably warm, not hot. Babies can't control their temperature.

□ Buy a non-slip mat for your shower or bathtub. Avoid bathing when alone in the house; it's reassuring to know someone's there to help in case you should slip.

"With my fourth baby I tried a complementary therapist to treat anxiety. She combined homeopathy, reflexology, and acupuncture in one session. I immediately felt an incredible peace and calm come over me ... I ended up having my first water birth and no stitches."

SUZANNE, MOTHER OF NIAMH, TARA, ALANNAH, AND CONNALL

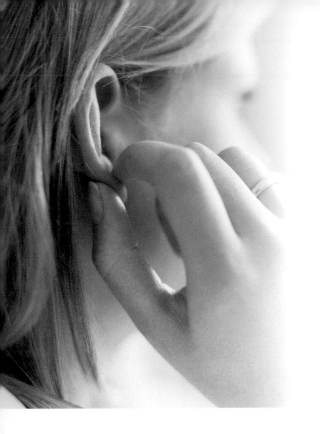

Make time, any time, to give yourself the opportunity of 5 to 10 minutes of instant relaxation. Try to fit any one of these quick-fix, do-it-yourself tips into your day.

1 This shiatsu massage technique helps to subdue the senses and stimulate the mental processes. Start by making up one of the aromatherapy pregnancy blends described on page 61 and massage it between your palms. Hold your palms over your nose and mouth and inhale. Then firmly press the fleshy part of both ears from the lower lobe upward. Repeat, then lightly press your fingertips along the brows, on to your temples, and along the nape of your neck.

TEN WAYS TO... *relax*

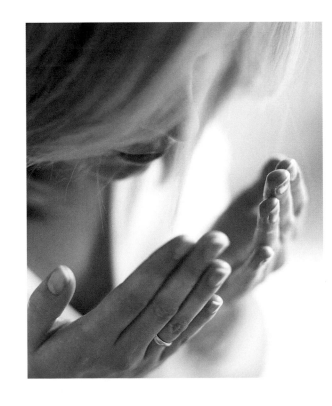

2 Place 3 to 5 drops of either lavender, rose, or geranium essential oil in a tissue, tuck it in your bra, and inhale deeply whenever you feel tense.

3 Deep breathing is not only for labor—it is the best way to calm your whole body. Sit upright in a comfortable chair, with your hands resting on your bump. Breathe in fully, count to two, then breathe out for a count of 6 at the same rate. Be aware of your hands rising and falling. Repeat 12 times.

4 Try color therapy to help you find the path to inner peace. Close your eyes and imagine your whole body bathed in a beautiful blue light or immersed in azure blue waters. Color therapists also recommend sleeping in blue nightclothes and between blue sheets, and keeping a low-wattage blue lightbulb illuminated throughout the night.

5 Give yourself a soothing back massage. Put two stress balls in a sock, spaced 2 in (5 cm) apart, and tie a rubber band around the open end. Lie on your back on the floor, placing one ball each side of the spine. Gently roll yourself up and down, focusing on tense areas.

6 Exercise your eyes, to make them feel brighter and relieve tension. Look straight ahead. Place your index fingers lengthwise under your eyebrows. Push up your eyebrows with your fingers and hold them firmly against the bone. Then close your eyelids very slowly, feeling the pull down from brow to lashes. Squeeze your eyelids together tightly. Hold for a count of five. Release for a count of five. Open your eyes and relax.

7 Lie back, place a pillow under your knees to take the strain off your back, and listen to a piece of music that helps you unwind. Plan to use this piece of music in labor if you can.

8 Relax in a soothing bath scented with 3 drops each of mandarin oil and rose oil. Add to still bath water and stir together before stepping in.

9 Treat your feet to a gentle, stroking massage. Prop up your feet and ask your partner to rub a little oil between his palms and then to place one hand flat on top of your foot and the other flat on the sole, and massage in a circular movement. He should place both thumbs under each of your feet in turn and rub each thumb along the length of the sole from heel to toes, and then massage each toe separately, gently pulling the toes to relax them further.

IO For 5–10 minutes of complete calm, sit comfortably with your shoulders down and relaxed, and your hands in your lap, palms facing up. Concentrate on the sensation in one hand and imagine it gradually getting warmer and warmer.

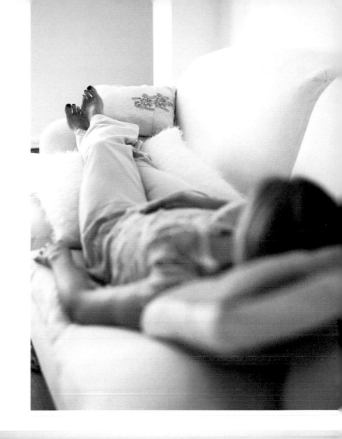

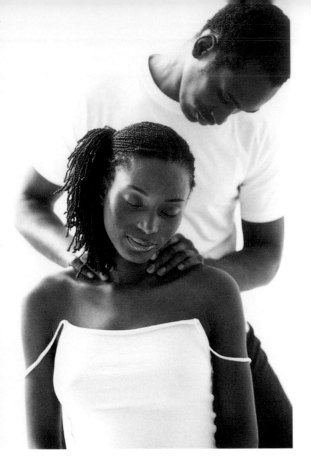

"I say go with the flow. If you feel you need an epidural and can't handle the pain, or are too tired, do it. You will have a happier birth experience—and better memories—if you trust your own instincts and do what makes you feel happiest."

CORINNA, MOTHER OF KATIE AND CHARLOTTE

counting down to labor

As you approach the end of the third trimester, there are some last-minute techniques that may help encourage the early onset of labor and make it more likely that you will have a more positive, active birth.

TIPS FOR A LESS STRESSFUL BIRTH

Leslie Spires, the head midwife for the Active Birth Centre at Queen Charlotte's & Chelsea Hospital in London, believes that there are several things you can do to make a rewarding birth more likely.

□ Prepare yourself. Knowledge can help to instill confidence if events take a different turn from what you had been expecting.

□ Have confidence. If women believe in themselves, they can have a very positive birth experience, even if they end up having to have a cesarean. A positive birth leads to a more positive attitude to motherhood.

□ Get support. Never underestimate the need to have the right person partnering you at the birth.

□ Choose your environment. Decide in advance whether you want to give birth at home, at a birth center, or in the hospital and work toward it. Even though you should be prepared for things to take a different course, you can have the birth you'd prefer.

ENCOURAGING LABOR

If you have reached your due date, or it is not far away, you may want to consider ways in which you can encourage labor to start and progress smoothly.

□ Drinking fresh raspberry leaf tea during the final four weeks of a pregnancy is believed to stimulate contractions of the uterus, helping to smooth the way and make labor easier.

□ Massaging and stimulating your nipples with a cream or oil may help to induce labor—as may sex at this time. Prostaglandins, substances in semen, are said to help dilate the cervix and are a well-known stimulus for labor once you have passed 40 weeks.

□ You may wish to consult an experienced reflexologist. Massage of specific zones in the feet is particularly effective at stimulating labor.

□ A soothing, soporific soak in a bath is still rated by midwives as one of the best natural methods of pain relief in the early stages of labor. Birthing pools are an increasingly popular way to control pain effectively in labor—most women find the warmth and buoyancy very comforting. In the last few weeks of pregnancy, try using your bathtub at home to relieve discomfort and aches and pains in much the same way.

□ During the final few weeks, add 5 drops of clary sage essential oil to your bath water—it is renowned for helping to stimulate uterine muscles.

□ Ask your partner to massage your aching back using gentle stroking movements—and without applying any pressure. Try straddling an upright chair or lying on your side using cushions for support.

COMPLEMENTARY PAIN RELIEF

There are several homeopathic remedies for different stages of labor. If homeopathy works for you, keep Caulophyllum for exhaustion and when labor is not progressing; Gelsemium for trembling and weakness; and Pulsatilla for indecisiveness or comfort. Pulsatilla is said to be effective in turning a breech baby (where the baby's feet rather than its head are presenting first).

Acupuncture and shiatsu are both known for their ability to block pain. If you want to use one of these techniques, arrange for a practitioner to be with you at the hospital and mention your wish in your birth plan.

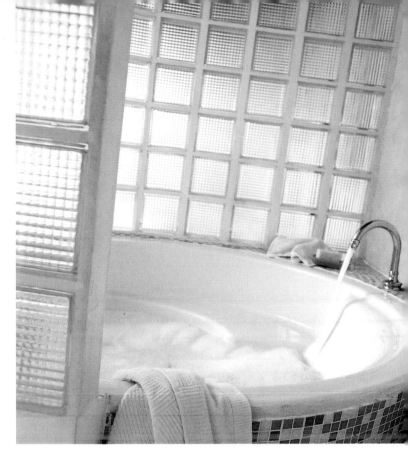

"I seemed to spend each of my three pregnancies in the bath, loving the way the water rippled around my ever-expanding bump. I would watch with love and amazement how the baby would practice stretching its limbs as if it was swimming."

JO, MOTHER OF OLIVIA, WILLIAM, AND PHOEBE

weeks 29–40 COUNTING DOWN TO LABOR

today, **hospitals** allow new **mothers** to leave earlier than ever before, **sometimes** within hours of the **birth**—but stay in for at **least** one **night** if you can

ready to go

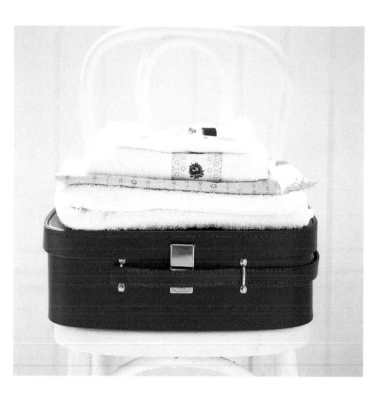

The big moment has almost arrived, and—unless you are intending to give birth at home—the time has come to think about what you and your baby will need during a short stay in the hospital.

WHAT YOU WILL NEED IN THE HOSPITAL

Despite the trend for new mothers to go home ever sooner after the birth (as long as there are no complications), I would recommend at least one overnight stay in hospital—simply for the support, especially if you are on your own at home. Expect to stay for several days after a cesarean.

Your hospital or midwife will probably provide a list of things to bring with you, but these are things mothers have recommended for your labor bag:

☐ A lightweight robe (not heavy terrycloth, which drags on newly sensitive nipples after birth).

☐ Lightweight, front-opening shirt.

☐ Stretchy pants that do not dig in anywhere.

☐ Plenty of maternity sanitary towels.

☐ Washbag with overnight essentials such as toothbrush, toothpaste, and soap.

☐ Antiseptic lavender essential oil. Add 6 drops to bath water to soothe and heal stitches.

☐ Slippers that you don't need to bend to put on.

☐ Bottle of spray water, since maternity wards are kept at a warm temperature.

☐ A cloth or soft sponge, which your partner can use to keep you cool in labor.

☐ Bottles of water and small cartons of fruit juice to keep up your fluid level, and drinking straws—so your birth partner can help you.

☐ A back massager tool to help to ease backache.

☐ On-site entertainment: relaxing music, hand-held games (such as Game Boy and Connect 4), books, word puzzles.

☐ Easy-to-eat snacks such as nuts and fruit to keep your energy up.

☐ Camera, loose change, list of telephone numbers to call after the birth.

for the baby

☐ Sleepsuit, scratch mitts, cardigan, hat.

☐ Cellular blanket.

☐ Gauze feeding squares.

☐ Baby carrier for going home.

"I remember so well, before the birth of my first child, not worrying about labor at all, but having sleepless nights about her as a teenager."

JO, MOTHER OF OLIVIA, WILLIAM, AND PHOEBE

becoming a parent

You have come this far, and have much farther to go together. It is a great test of your partnership. Someone small needs you both now—to feel safe, loved, and nurtured in every way.

RE-LEARNING LIFE FROM THE BEGINNING

Jim and I knew when we wanted children. We had reached a time in our lives when everything was ticking along fine, but there seemed to be no real point. Then along came these little innocents with no preconceived ideas, who learned everything from new, experiencing it with the kind of energy and enthusiasm you want to bottle up and preserve forever.

Becoming a parent lets you re-learn life from the beginning: enjoying measureless merriment in simple games, appreciating the beauty of nature as your child buries its nose in a flower—a happy smile, a first hug, total unconditional love. There is nothing to beat being a parent—but it is not without its challenges. You are embarking on probably the biggest upheaval in your life so far. A new baby has been described as "a cataclysmic intrusion on a previously pleasant existence."

SLEEP DEPRIVATION

Be prepared for the fact that you are going to be tired—it is simply a fact. Sleep deprivation is the single worst torture known to man—and woman. You may turn out to be lucky, but don't expect it. This is another good reason for getting as much rest as possible before the birth. Partners suffer from tiredness as well as new mothers. They get disturbed at night, then have to go to work next day, and smile supportively while everyone asks how *you* are. Resentment can easily creep in, which is why it's important to communicate with each other, to share all the pleasures of your new baby as well as the new routine, and involve your partner all the more.

CHANGING RELATIONSHIPS

You, at least initially, will have a much closer bond with the baby simply because you are its main carer and nurturer. A new father may resent the attention given to this new being—perhaps seeing a new side to your personality—which makes everything seem tenser than you might have imagined at this emotional time. It is easily done. We can lose sight of our selves and our relationship—the whole reason the baby is here in the first place—because we are busy putting the baby first.

So, above all, remember each other. If you are fortunate enough to have a good relationship, make it stronger and try devoting quality time to yourselves as a couple whenever you get the chance.

there is **nothing** to **beat** being

a **parent**—you just **might** have

to **remind** yourself of

the **fact** from **time** to time

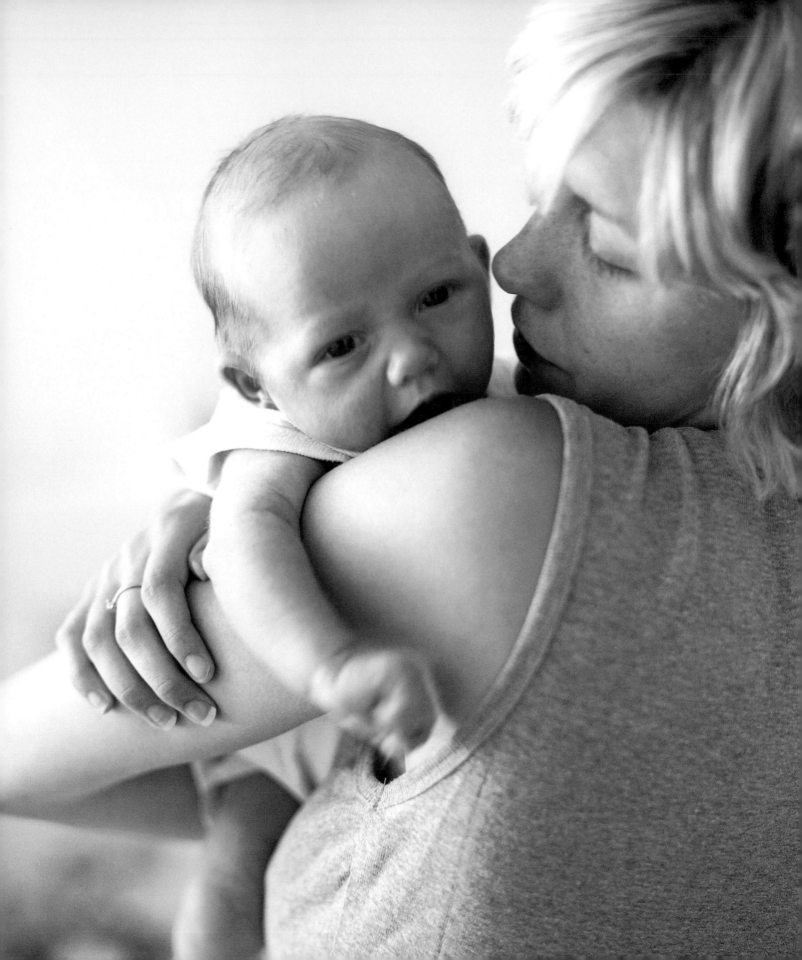

the birth and beyond

You are on the brink. This is what your body has always been meant to do. You may feel anxious about things unknown, but go with the rhythm. Your body will do what it has to do. You simply need to keep mind and body as one. Trust your instincts, listen to your body, and above all, relax.

giving birth

Suddenly you are very much aware what all those relaxation tips, comfortable positions, and breathing techniques are for. Your body is doing what it can do naturally—and the more in tune, relaxed, and focused on the event you are, the more positive it will be.

THE STAGES OF BIRTH

The birthing process consists of three stages, which your health practitioner will guide you through. The first stage is the longest, averaging between 2 and 12 hours.

the first stage

The uterus contracts at regular intervals—though contractions sometimes come and go—until the cervix dilates, or opens, to 4 in (10 cm) in diameter, at which point the baby's head can pass through. The first stage ends in transition. This is usually a short but powerful sequence of contractions that dilate the cervix to its full extent. Your midwife may tell you to pant through transition; you may feel nauseous, shaky, and irritable.

the second stage

This stage involves the actual birth of the baby and is much quicker than the first, though intense. With the cervix fully dilated, you push your baby through the cervix, pelvic canal, and finally out through the vagina.

the third stage

The third stage is the delivery of the placenta shortly after the delivery of the baby. Final contractions push the placenta out—like a mini birth. To avoid any complications, it is important for the medical staff to make sure the placenta is delivered intact

AM I IN LABOR?

There are several signs that you are in labor.

□ You experience regular contractions. Contractions may come and go in intensity and last for a whole day before things really get started.

□ You get a "show," where the protective mucus plug comes away from the cervix and is expelled from the vagina. It may be bloodstained and occur either during the first stage or a few days before contractions start.

□ Your waters break. You will experience this as either a warm trickle or a gush of clear fluid, and you may even feel a little "pop." Consult your health practitioner if it happens. There are two types of "waters"—the fore-waters (the main amount of amniotic fluid) and the hind-waters (a small amount). If only the hind-waters break, labor is less likely to follow fast, but you should still consult your doctor since you may risk infection.

for some **women**, the pain of **labor** seems just like **backache**; for others, it's a **mild** cramp like menstrual **pain**; and for **others**, it's a strong **contraction**

> "Getting mothers to relax in a birthing environment is vital; otherwise, anxiety builds up and contractionsmay slow down—then pain relief is required and more intervention often follows."

LESLIE SPIRES, HEAD MIDWIFE, QUEEN CHARLOTTE'S
& CHELSEA HOSPITAL ACTIVE BIRTH CENTRE, LONDON

WHAT DO CONTRACTIONS FEEL LIKE?

We all experience pain differently. For some, the pain of early labor may resemble backache or a mild cramp like menstrual pain; for others, it is a series of full-on strong contractions from the beginning.

For many women, labor starts gently with mild contractions, each lasting 20 to 30 seconds at intervals of around 10 to 20 minutes. Gradually, the contractions become longer, stronger, and more frequent, until they last almost a whole minute and occur every 2 to 3 minutes, each with a distinct peak of intensity in the middle. This is established labor. Other women may not get regular contractions without help (usually in the form of an injection of oxytocin). Others may go straight into strong regular contractions. Every variation can be described as "normal."

A hospital will not usually expect to see you until your contractions are 5 minutes apart. If you can wait this long, you can do most of your relaxation and breathing exercises in the comfort of your own home. Remember that tension can shut down your body's natural mechanisms—so practice those relaxation techniques. A bath is a great place to be in early labor. Add soothing essential oils such as lavender, geranium, rose, and neroli to keep you feeling calm.

HOW DO I KNOW WHEN IT IS TIME TO PUSH?

Your health practitioner will help you control your breathing and pushing so that each effort brings the baby nearer to being born. The second stage often lasts between 20 minutes and 1 hour, and involves a series of about 10 to 15 big pushes. The urge to push the baby out feels exactly the same as the need to empty your bowels—and it is exactly that bearing-down action that you need to replicate now with each contraction.

Your health practitioner can gauge how effectively you are pushing. If you have had an epidural (which numbs the pelvic area and the legs), all you need to do is to push when you are told to by the doctor, using your back passage.

Do what comes naturally. Try to avoid holding your breath, which can make you feel exhausted, and relax your body as you push. Being tense only works against the natural instinct to push. Go with the whole sensation to help your body push the baby out.

CAN I COPE WITH THE PAIN?

Be realistic. Don't delude yourself one way or the other about the pain of childbirth. Be prepared to have pain relief if you can't cope—but, equally, be prepared to cope better than you have anticipated. Unlike the pain of an injury, the pain of birth is a positive pain—a pain all the same, but a sign that something is being achieved. Think of it confidently as a challenge rather than something to fear or something to ignore.

Active birth centers pride themselves on their laidback approach to childbirth. "Midwives themselves are more relaxed about their own practice," says Leslie Spires. "There's none of the rigid routines and starched uniforms of the traditional maternity ward. The environment is geared toward a more positive, natural birth—and what is birth if not natural?"

preparing to deal with pain

What are your plans for labor and birth? Indeed, have you made any?
"Preparation is everything when it comes to the birth," says Leslie Spires.
"If you have a good idea about what's meant to happen, how to use
your breathing, and how you would ideally like the baby delivered, you
will ultimately be more in control."

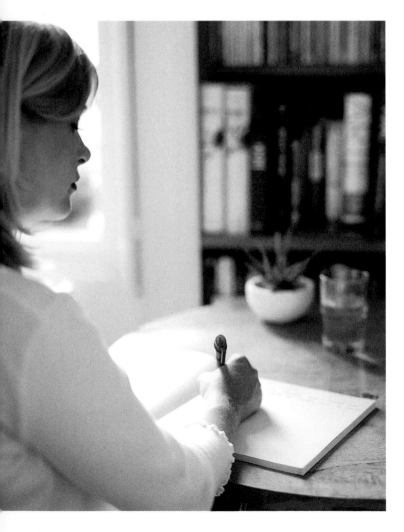

AN ACTIVE BIRTH

A woman who wants to deliver her baby as naturally
as possible, has no known complications (such as pre-
eclampsia), and does not require an induction, is a
suitable candidate for what is called an "active" birth. In
these circumstances, where the need for intervention is
clearly less likely, the woman is supported by a midwife
and simply allowed to get on with it. However, if the
active birth center in question is attached to a hospital,
the woman has the reassurance that there is a medical
team on hand should she or her baby need them.

Labor is a physical task. It is exhausting—and, if you
are tense and rigid, it is all the harder to cope with.
In labor, when your uterus contracts strongly, other
muscles in your body join in. But when you relax, the
contractions work more effectively and your body's
natural painkilling hormones flow.

"I've witnessed many women in labor who have
regular contractions that stop the moment their
partner leaves the room," says Leslie Spires. "It's your
body's natural safety mechanism to shut down when
you don't feel at ease. Then, the moment the partner
returns, everything switches back on. This simply
highlights how important it is to relax in order for
everything to get going."

YOUR BIRTH PLAN

It is helpful to make a birth plan, detailing the kind of birth you would prefer to have. Ask your health practitioner for advice. Be as open-minded and realistic as possible when making the plan, but stress things that matter to you—you might have strong views about being monitored, having a water birth, or having your baby delivered on your tummy.

WHAT A PAIN

There is increasing pressure on women to give birth with minimal pain relief. An active birth—in which you are encouraged to move around freely, unconstrained by monitors, allowing your body to behave naturally—is considered to be a more positive introduction into the world for your baby. And while there is obviously labor pain—greater for some women than others—it is a power pain, something to take control of and use to push the baby out.

Labor pain is an experience, one that in hindsight may seem something that was not to be missed. But hindsight is all well and good. At the time, you need to feel that you can cope. And if coping means having more pain relief—in the form of gas and air, pethidine, or an epidural, for example—it is still a positive birth, for you are calling the shots.

If you can take the pain, childbirth is an amazing sensation. If you can't, it is still an amazing experience. And by making sure your baby is born directly onto your tummy (or into your arms after a cesarean), that the first suckle from your breast is within minutes (even if you don't continue to breastfeed later), you have still had a positive birth. It is your decision.

RELAX AND BREATHE

This is the moment when birthing partners really come into their own. In the midst of everything you are having to do and not do (push—don't push; pant—breathe slowly), you need someone calm who is there for you and can remind you how to breathe (as learned at prenatal classes).

Deep breathing is a known form of relaxation, and is the single best way to control your body and release tension that can otherwise hinder the birthing process.

Your aim when breathing calmly and slowly is to drop your shoulders, open up your hands, and relax your jaw and teeth. Visualize easy, slow breathing, emphasizing the outward breath, with a slight pause before you breathe in again. Choose any one of the positions on pages 124–25 whenever you need to relax—even when you are not in labor.

At the start of each contraction, take a deep breath, breathing out slowly as it peaks in the middle, inhaling slowly as the pain subsides. (During any physical exercise—especially labor—you should always exhale slowly when you are making an effort and inhale when you are recovering.) Between contractions, breathe slowly and deeply. When contractions are longer, you will need to take a few smaller, short, shallow breaths to get you over the peak.

other things your birthing partner can do
□ Provide encouragement. "You're doing brilliantly" can sound so reassuring on the crest of a contraction.
□ Lend you a hand to hold.
□ Massage and soothe you.
□ Comfort you with a cool, damp facecloth, crushed ice, or a sip of water or juice.

midwives regard **massage** of the mother's **lower back** in **labor** as an excellent **natural** method of pain relief

Natural herbal extracts, homeopathic remedies, massage, and aromatherapy can all play a role in making labor easier. And, although what works for one woman may not work for all, this is a good time to seek advice from other new mothers about their experiences and the techniques they used to speed things along on the day.

1 Drinking raspberry leaf tea in the last six weeks of pregnancy is believed to help tone the uterus and soften the membranes, and to promote speedier dilation of the cervix during labor.

TEN WAYS TO... *ease labor*

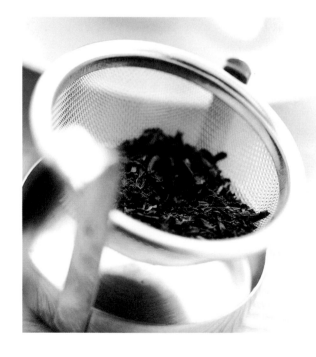

2 Herbal tinctures such as blue cohosh, black cohosh, and mugwort are recommended by leading herbalists as natural aids to establishing stronger, more regular contractions—but any of these can all be dangerous if misused during labor, so it is important to make sure the person administering these herbs knows what he or she is doing.

3 Bach Flower Rescue Remedy can be taken during labor to induce calm and make you feel more in control of what's happening. Put four drops on the tongue or in a glass of water.

4 To get the contractions going once you are past your due date, have a bath using clary sage. This should be used at no other time during pregnancy.

5 Choose homeopathy for various stages of childbirth. If contractions become ineffectual, try Pulsatilla 30C. For pain relief, try Caulophyllum 30C (or 60C from your practitioner).

6 When things simply get to be too much, learn to detach yourself from it all and escape to the sanctity of your bathroom. Pack some music tapes, essential oils, and other comforting items in your labor bag, in case it all takes longer than you had planned.

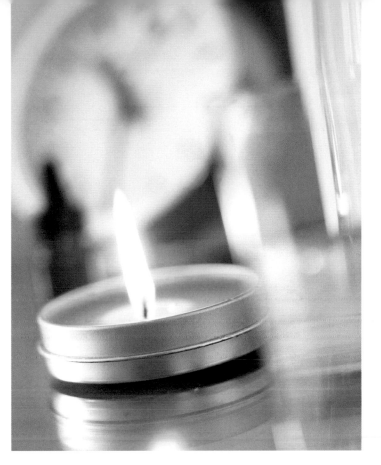

7 Play relaxing music and light a mood enhancing scented candle. I gave birth to a relaxation tape called Temple of the Forest by David Naegle—all twittering tropical birds of paradise and waterfalls—and played it in my baby's bedroom for the following six months after birth. Today, aged eight, she still pauses and stops to listen whenever I play it.

8 Scent your room and the delivery suite with lavender essential oil. It is relaxing and restorative, and balances out any anxieties or fear of pain. "I used my lavender oil burner at each of my children's births. It really helps." Esther, mother of Tess, Fay, and Claus.

9 Ask your partner to give you a soothing back rub with a massage tool that really feels like strong fingers kneading your shoulders. Make up your Relax Blend (see page 61) and use it in labor. Rub it on Ayurvedic vital points on the body (called marmas) that promote sleep and deep relaxation, on the center of the forehead and the back of the neck.

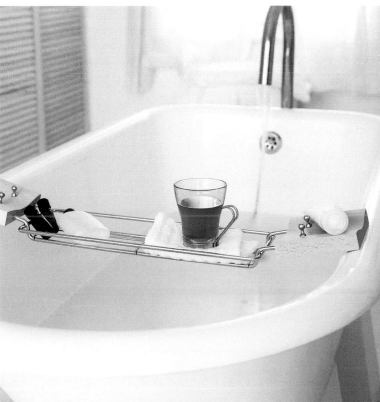

10 Think about using a TENS machine, which works by blocking the pain messages to the brain, almost numbing the effect. This was all I used during the first stage of labor. The pain was there, but I focused on the annoyingly tingly sensation in my back instead, which really worked.

positions for comfort in labor

To help you feel more confident and in control during labor, there are a number of positions for the different stages that are worth knowing about and practising in advance.

TO RELIEVE PAIN IN THE FIRST STAGE

The early part of labor is the time to feel relaxed and try out a variety of positions that instinctively feel good to you. Ideally, you should keep moving between contractions—being upright whenever possible means that you are using gravity to encourage the baby's natural descent. Move into a position you like when a contraction starts and breath calmly through it.

One way to calm yourself during contractions is to visualize your baby inside your tummy and imagine what is happening as it passes through the birth canal.

MOVING AROUND IN LABOR

If you are attached to a fetal monitor—which is a near certainty if you have experienced any problems in pregnancy—this will restrict your movement, since you will be less able to walk around freely in labor.

It is worth finding out in advance your hospital's policy on monitoring, since it may well affect your birth plan; some hospitals monitor constantly as a matter of routine.

In general, there should be no need for you to remain on a monitor if your baby is not in distress. However, if you have been induced or there is cause for concern, you may need to be monitored throughout.

STANDING

Standing up and leaning forward against a wall or against your partner can help to stimulate contractions and encourage your baby's descent. Try circling your hips or rock them from side to side in this position to relieve the pain. If you are leaning like this against a wall, ask your partner to massage your lower back to soothe pain effectively.

ROCKING

Kneeling on all fours and rocking your hips backward and forward during each contraction will help you to move rhythmically through the pain. When the pain gets very intense, you may prefer to kneel forward, with your bottom up and head resting on the floor.

KNEELING

Kneeling down with your bump supported by a beanbag, a birthing ball, or a big pile of cushions is a very comfortable position, especially if you can get some rest during mild contractions.

LYING

Lying down on your side with your bump supported by pillows and cushions and one leg raised is a comfortable position when you are tired.

TO PUSH YOUR BABY OUT

"We actively discourage women in labor from lying flat on their backs," says Nicky Wales, a midwife at Queen Charlotte's & Chelsea Active Birth Centre. "Leaning forward is the best position, or on all fours—you can reduce the likelihood of tearing, and very few women have an active birth in the bed."

staying upright or leaning

Standing upright or leaning against a wall are also good positions for delivery, making pushing easier. There is a straightforward explanation for why it is harder to push when you are lying on your back: you are pushing in the wrong direction.

squatting or kneeling on all fours

These are natural positions for labor because they use gravity to aid in the birthing process. Squatting opens your pelvis as widely as possible, yet relieves pressure at the same time. Supporting your weight on your partner's arms—or on one of your midwife's arms and one of your birthing partner's—place your feet hip width apart; with each contraction, bend your knees and open your pelvis.

sitting

Sitting is another common position for birth. Practice sitting up, propped against a pile of cushions, with your knees bent and apart. Tuck your head into your chest.

delivered lying on you, your **newborn baby** can enjoy the **warmth** of your **body** and the **comfort** of your **heartbeat**—familiar features of the past nine months

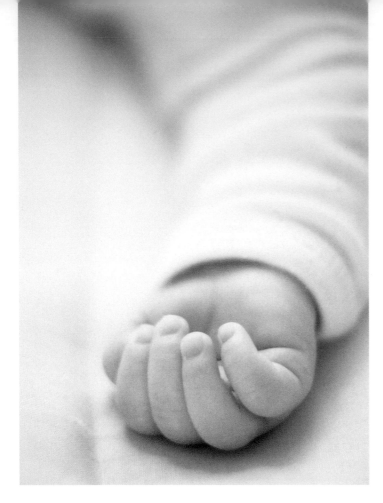

"My lavender baths were the one thing that kept me going. I had used lavender during each of my pregnancies, used it in labor and immediately after giving birth. I always associate its aroma with peace and tranquility at home—and, whenever I smell lavender now, I can instantly recollect each special moment of birth."

LIZ, MOTHER OF LILY, GUY, GABRIELLE, AND CHRISTIAN

your moment arrives

Such excitement. The midwife can touch and see the crown of your baby's head. It has passed beyond the cervix into the vagina—and a new child is on its way into the world.

DELIVERING THE BABY

Any medical staff who are in the delivery room will prepare for the birth by putting on gloves, laying out sterile equipment, and carefully washing the perineum and the area between your legs with an antiseptic solution.

Your health practitioner will encourage you to push. This is the time to feel your body doing its thing, while trusting yourself and the experienced staff around you. Once the head has been delivered, you will probably be asked to pant while it is gently eased out, then give another push to ease the baby's body out, too.

If the baby is delivered onto your body, it means that you and your child have immediate contact. The baby will be covered with a white coating called vernix that protects its skin while it is in the amniotic fluid, and his or her eyes may be a little puffy. The medical staff will want to whisk away the baby for weighing and checking that everything is fine. But try to seize those few moments together, which are emotionally uplifting for all three of you. If you can latch your baby onto your breast at this moment, it is a great way to establish a sucking technique as early as possible.

BIRTHS THAT NEED HELP

Episiotomy enlarges the vaginal opening to allow the baby's head to be delivered more easily. Performed under local anesthetic, it involves making a small cut that is stitched up afterward. The procedure should be explained beforehand and not be given routinely. Alternatively, you may tear to some degree. It may be a fine line between having an episiotomy and not having one, but an experienced practitioner will advise.

When the mother is too tired or unable to push (perhaps following an epidural), forceps may be used to clamp around the baby's head to protect it and ease it out. Ventouse—a suction cap that's applied to the baby's head—may be used instead of forceps. The use of either instrument can distort the baby's head shape for a few days. If the birth has put great pressure on your baby's head, consider seeking cranial osteopathy from a professional practitioner.

A baby whose bottom or feet present for delivery before its head is known as a breech. Some breech babies are born by cesarean section; in other cases, the baby's head may have to be helped out with forceps.

A cesarean section, in which the baby is delivered through the lower abdomen, is either planned (elective) or may be chosen at the last minute in response to complications such as fetal distress. If you need a cesarean, stay positive. Focus on the thought that it's not just an operation, it's a new addition to the family.

STILLBIRTH

Nothing can prepare either of you for the loss of your long-awaited baby. Grief takes many forms, but talking openly to your partner, close friends, or a counselor will help you adjust and come to terms over time with your immense loss. Do try to see, hold, and smell your baby. Memories are everything.

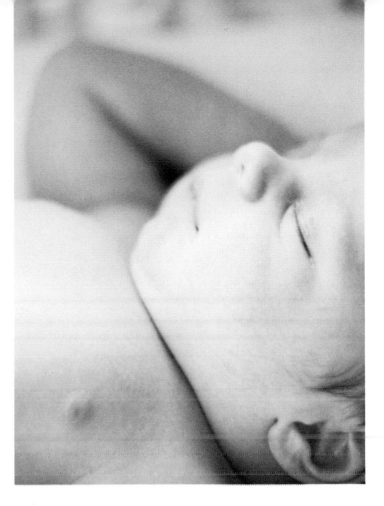

"During the birth I could get no relief from constant contractions. I needed gas and air, but it didn't seem to do much for me. Suddenly it was as if I'd pushed through a 'ceiling of pain.' I was above it all and it was amazing. In 20 minutes my son was born, but I'll never forget that out-of-body feeling."

SUZANNE, MOTHER OF NIAMH, TARA, ALANNAH, AND CONNAL

sea salt is fantastic in a **bath** after labor to help

to **soothe** and **heal** bruises and stitches—add

two pounds to the **water** and sit in it for 20 minutes

"Wear only pajamas for the first three weeks. You've just been through a life-changing experience that is both physically and emotionally draining. Of course, everyone wants to visit—but if you wear pajamas it subtly says, 'Be gentle with me,' and makes them realize instinctively that you need nurturing."

LIZ, MOTHER OF LILY, GUY, GABRIELLE, AND CHRISTIAN

after the birth

Don't stop taking care of yourself now that your baby is here. There are many helpful remedies and techniques to heal you and promote wellbeing for you both.

RECOVERING FROM THE BIRTH

Give yourself plenty of time to recover. Many new mothers expect to return to normal quickly, but this is a time to nurture both yourself and your baby. Remember the advice: "You can only be as good as a mother as you are good at mothering yourself."

In birth-proud nations such as many in Africa, the family takes over and a new mother is barely allowed to move. She stays in bed feeding herself and her baby. Modern life in the developed world places demands upon us, but don't let yourself get stressed out. Forget the washing and cleaning, ignore the office—and, at least for the first four weeks, accept every offer of help.

To help to heal stitches and keep the pelvic area free from infection, bathe regularly in a bath containing five drops of antiseptic and antiviral lavender essential oil. Ice cubes wrapped in a clean towel and held against the stitches help to reduce bruising, as do arnica homeopathic tablets 30C and arnica cream—but take care not to use arnica cream on broken skin.

Women with sore, cracked nipples should try using an herbal tincture made from hypericum and calendula (called Hypercal). Alternate it with calendula cream or chamomile ointment between feeds for three to four days—no longer or your nipples may become "soggy." Wipe your nipples clean before feeding because some preparations contain peanut oil, which may lead to a nut allergy in sensitive babies.

Cranial osteopathy helps to rebalance the body and relieve stress and tension by gently manipulating the bones of the skull, which then boosts the nervous system. The technique is very gentle and can be used to treat babies, too, most commonly in cases of colic.

Put 3 drops of relaxing Roman chamomile essential oil in your bathtub and share a bath with your baby. Some pediatricians advise women against wearing perfume while breastfeeding because it may interfere with the baby's sense of smell, but a few drops of perfume in the bathwater will soothe a restless babe and unify both you and your baby in your scent.

"I tried breastfeeding for four weeks, but my little boy didn't gain huge amounts of weight. He was always hungry and never satisfied—so I soon got tired and stressed because of it. I began topping him up with formula milk for three feeds in the day, and he immediately became the happy, contented baby I'd expected."

SHARON, MOTHER OF HAMISH

feeding for two...means you, too

You will probably have given plenty of thought to how you will feed your baby. With many experts touting the virtues of breast milk over formula, it is hard not to feel pressurized, but whether or not to breastfeed is a personal decision that you alone should make.

THE PROS AND CONS OF BREASTFEEDING

Breast milk gives your baby special nutrients that help develop its immune system, guards against infection, and may offer protection from SIDS. Breastfeeding also creates an initial closeness between mother and child through skin-to-skin contact, and may help you to regain your figure by stimulating the release of oxytocin (which prompts the uterus to return to its ordinary size). Breast milk is free, available whenever you need it, and can be expressed into a bottle using a pump.

But a stressed mother makes for a stressed baby. Sore nipples can crack, bleed, and feel very painful. If you believe that you are producing insufficient milk for your baby, it leads to worry, which leads to even less milk—in a vicious cycle that is hard to break without complete rest and carefully monitored fluids and food. Likewise, too much milk (spurting everywhere uncomfortably) leads to stress at a time when you should be cuddling, snuggling, and happy.

A happy mother is what your baby needs most. Don't breastfeed because you feel you ought to. It is a beautiful thing to experience when it settles down after a couple of weeks—and it does. But if it does not work for you, don't feel guilty about it.

BREASTFEEDING TIPS

□ The first milk at birth is colostrum, which contains vital antibodies for your baby's health. By the third or fourth day, your breasts will become hot and enlarged (engorgement), then your breast milk "comes in."

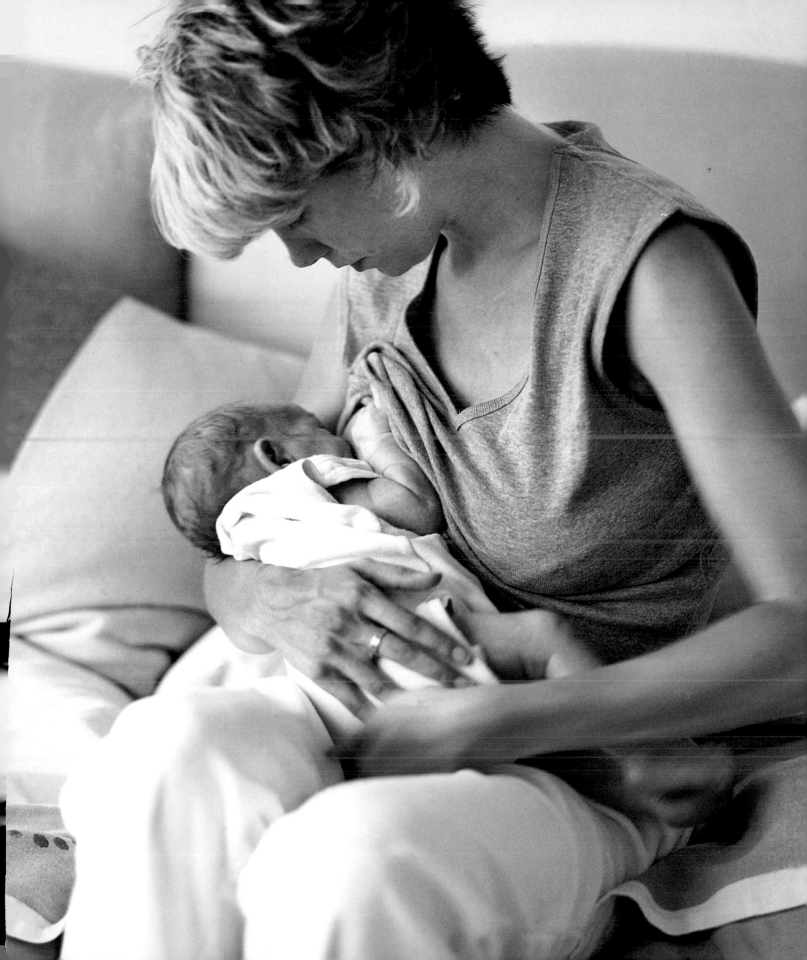

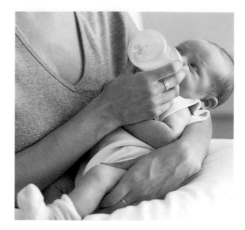

"I breastfed each of my three children for six months. There were highs and lows—times when I thought I'd eaten all the wrong things because one child wouldn't stop bringing it all back or another was colicky. But I'd go through it all over again, and it became easier with each baby."

MARTHA, MOTHER OF HARRIET, CHARLOTTE, AND TILDA

□ When your breasts become engorged, alternate a hot and cold cloth dipped in a bowl of water (add lavender oil if you wish) to relieve discomfort. Feeding is the best way to ease engorgement fast. Regular feeding also helps prevent blocked milk ducts. Express excess milk and massage your breasts in a hot bath.

□ Positioning is important for successful breastfeeding. Support your back at all times. Sit comfortably and place a pillow on your lap to help raise the baby's mouth in line with your breast. Gently turn the baby's whole body to face your tummy and cradle its head on the crook of your arm. A swaddled baby feels more content and secure, and is easier for you to maneuver from one breast to the other while you are getting used to the technique. Gently squeeze the areola (the dark circle around the nipple) so that its shape matches the width of your baby's mouth, and place it all in the baby's mouth. If your baby takes only the nipple, it will hurt in no time at all. To make sure the entire areola enters the baby's mouth, it may help to spread the first finger and thumb of your spare hand and lightly place these under the breast, which allows you to support the breast and direct the nipple more accurately. Practice this position until you feel more confident about feeding. Once your baby latches on effectively, try feeding while lying on your side (useful at night in bed) or with the baby held under one arm like a football.

□ If your nipples are very sore, you can express milk for a few days to relieve them and help them heal. "Chamomile is good for calming mother and baby," says Glenda Taylor, "and can be used safely in a very light dilution for healing sore nipples. Either put a few drops in water and bathe the nipples, add a few drops to a base lotion or oil, or use a chamomile ointment."

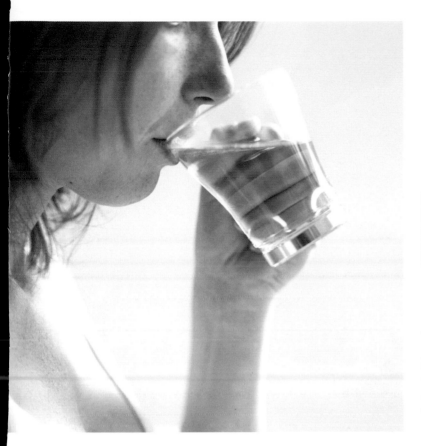
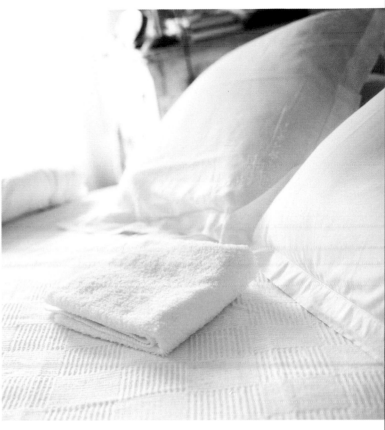

□ Fennel essential oil helps to stimulate the hormones responsible for lactation. Put a few drops in the bath or diffuse it in a vaporizer. Drinking fennel tea helps to boost milk flow and milk production.

□ Keep milk supply and energy up by getting plenty of rest, eating well, and drinking plenty of fluids. Drink a glass of water whenever you are feeding.

□ Choose healthy one-handed snacks so you can eat while rocking, winding, soothing, or feeding your baby—for example, hummus and pita bread, ready-prepared crudites and dips, slices of quiche, and small open sandwiches. Ask your partner to prepare some easy snacks that you can eat with one hand and a pitcher of a fruit smoothie (see page 66 for recipes).

□ Drink chamomile tea and offer a teaspoon of chamomile tea in place of water to a baby with colic symptoms; it may help to relax its digestive system. At some times of the day (especially if it is hot), you may find that your breast milk feeds rather than quenches a thirst. The best way to test this is to touch your baby's fontanel on the crown. If it is slightly dipped, this usually indicates mild dehydration. A spoonful of cooled boiled water usually balances this out, and your baby may seem happier, though some breastfeeding experts say that breast milk gives a baby everything it needs.

□ Breastfeeding does not automatically help you lose your pregnancy weight. It helps the uterus regain its shape, but if you crave high-carbohydrate and sugary foods, you are likely to gain weight. Eat a well-balanced diet and you won't be too disappointed. But don't diet while breastfeeding. You both need nourishment now.

□ If you are worried that you are producing insufficient milk, you can try to improve your milk flow using the homeopathic remedy Ignatia 30C.

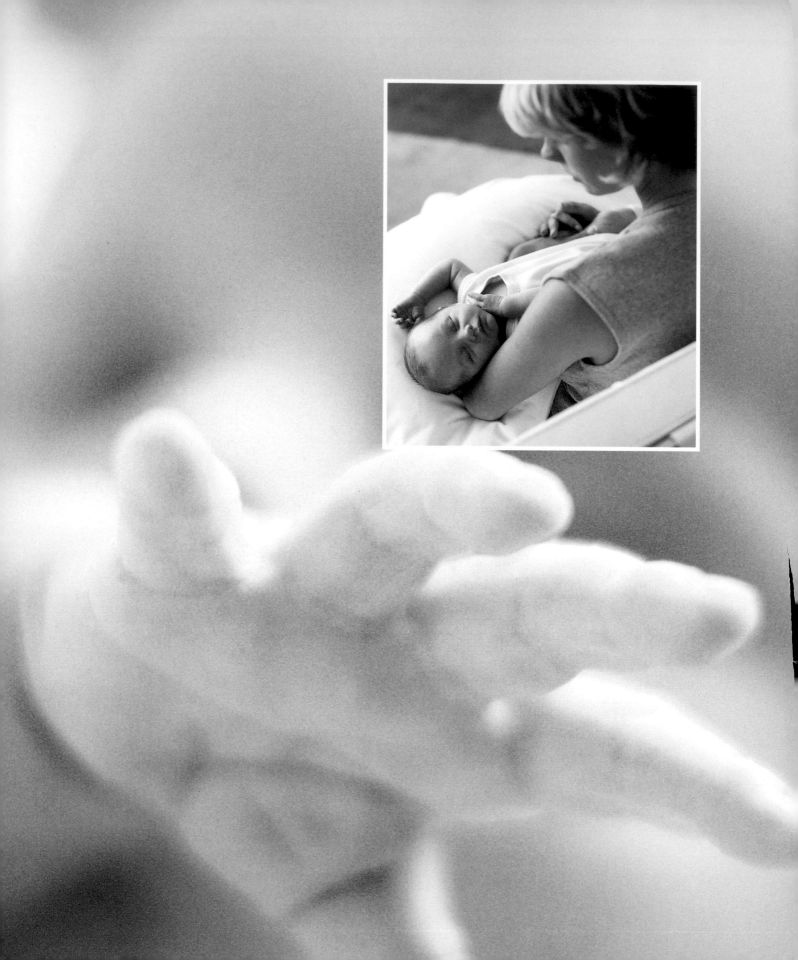

how are you feeling?

Are you elated? Are you full of immense love and wonderment at this tiny being that you have just brought into the world? Capture all the positive emotions of this marvelous experience—they will help you cope brilliantly over the next few months.

FLUCTUATING EMOTIONS

Caring for a new baby is exhilarating but exhausting, and more stressful than you might first imagine—with lack of sleep, anxiety, and postnatal changes to your hormone levels leading to tiredness and tears. It is estimated that in the first week after the birth three out of four new mothers experience mood swings or "baby blues" to some extent, but it often lasts as long as two weeks.

Postnatal depression is more severe—and, although it is also triggered by hormonal changes and fatigue, other emotional and financial strains may play a part. If you find that prolonged feelings of anxiety, fretfulness, despondency, or lack of interest in your baby persist, consult your doctor. The more that becomes known about postnatal depression, the more doctors too readily categorize hormonal and emotional new mothers as depressive. Always talk about how you feel with those around you who know you best. Let them help you determine how deep your feelings go.

REMEDIES FOR HORMONAL PROBLEMS

Whether you are suffering from serious postnatal depression or mild mood swings, there are things you can do to make yourself feel better.

☐ Fragrant jasmine and clary sage aromatherapy essential oils both have antidepressant properties that boost relaxation and may help to lift postnatal depression. Add 6 drops of either to a warm bath and relax in it, diffuse them in the air, or add 3 drops of either to a tissue and inhale throughout each day. See an aromatherapist for a more intensive treatment.

☐ Cranial osteopathy is said to release strain patterns caused by childbirth that affect the mood.

☐ Consider your diet. Foods rich in magnesium, zinc, and vitamins B2 and B6 may help to normalize hormone levels, while unrefined carbohydrates, such as wholewheat bread, and protein help to maintain your blood sugar levels to prevent mood swings.

☐ Try visualization. Imagine a positive scene—it could be something as simple as your baby feeding contentedly. One study of new mothers reported that most produced over 60 percent more breast milk after listening to a 20-minute guided relaxation tape.

SEXUAL FEELINGS

Isn't it strange how your newborn seems to stir and squawk every time your partner puts his arms around you in bed? Many postnatal counselors believe that almost half of first-time mothers have no sexual relations with their partner for between six months and a year after the birth. If you are breastfeeding, the chances are there is only one reason why you are awake in the night.

The modern, child-centered approach to parenting, coupled with the fact that women are encouraged to breastfeed for as long as possible, often means that your sex life is put on the back burner. Womanly and motherly don't readily go hand in hand. Leaking breasts and sleep deprivation may not make you feel much like

135

a love goddess, but try not to abandon one of nature's greatest relaxants. You and your partner will both need to make more of an effort now that someone small demands most of your energy. Try setting aside some quality time for each other. Why not arrange a night away, leaving bottles (breast or formula milk—the odd night will do no harm) with a trusted sitter. Find ways to be intimate other than through intercourse. Some women fear that intimacy will lead to sex, so they withdraw physical affection entirely, which then upsets their partner. Talking about it can lessen the problem.

reasons why we go off sex (partners: please read)
□ At the end of a day spent attending to the needs of a demanding baby, we are exhausted—with the result that the needs of our partner are put on hold.
□ The release of prolactin while breastfeeding depresses the mother's libido.
□ Women associate sex with pregnancy, and the last thing you may want right now is to get pregnant again.

RETURNING TO YOUR ORDINARY SIZE
Straight after the birth, it can be startling to see your now empty "bump" looking sloppy and squashy. It will start to shrink over the next two weeks, and by six weeks you should be near your prepregnancy size. You may wish to bear in mind that some private hospitals can include a tummy tuck with a cesarean if requested.

EXERCISE
The kind of exercises to focus on for the first couple of weeks are your pelvic-floor exercises (see pages 68–69) and some abdominal exercises (unless you have had a cesarean, in which case you will have to take it easier for the first six weeks). There is nothing to stop you from doing aerobic classes the day you come back from the hospital—but ideally wait until the lochia (the site of the placenta on the uterine wall) has stopped bleeding, which can take up to two weeks.

Try learning some exercises you can do at home. Steps on the stairs, yoga, Pilates, tai chi are all good for mind and body. Buy a soft floor mat. Practice "peekabo sit-ups" with your baby on your lap, or "the buggy run"—brisk walking for more than 20 minutes in the park. If you do an intensive workout, bear in mind that exercise increases the amount of lactic acid in breast milk, making it taste sourer to a baby. Plan exercise so you don't need to feed immediately afterward.

RE-ESTABLISHING DIGESTIVE RHYTHMS
Your first bowel movement may not occur for days after the birth. The reason may be as much psychological as physiological: you have just used those very muscles to push a baby out—why would you want to go there again? Also, the area is probably quite bruised and sore from stitches. Eat plenty of high-fiber foods and try those that have a natural laxative effect such as prunes. Ideally, you should have your first bowel movement by the seventh day.

Urinating is not usually a problem after the birth, except that it may sting where you have been newly stitched. If it feels very uncomfortable, sit in a shallow bath of water and urinate into the water to dilute the effect. Remember to drink plenty of fluids—especially water. This will help to dilute your urine from within.

if you find that your **libido** seems to have reached **an all-time low**, try setting aside some quality time to spend with **your partner**

"I must admit that I felt as if my body was no longer my own after the birth. It was uncomfortable to sit for a couple of days, but I had my baby to focus on and soon got back to normal—well, pretty much."

HELEN, MOTHER OF CARRIE AND TOM

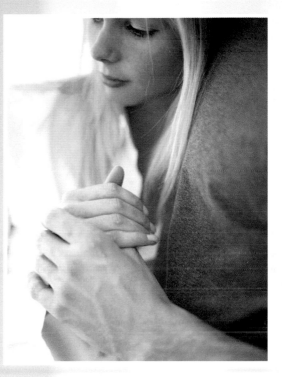

you matter, too

Motherhood will change you in many ways. You will certainly become less self-obsessed than you were in your childless days, when you had all that time for you and your partner. And there's a lot of extra work. But your quality of life matters, because you matter. You have a new responsibility to keep yourself feeling happy, positive, and healthy. So create time for you.

LOOKING GOOD

Start by going to the hairdresser. Get a new style or cut plenty off (a short style is often easier to manage). Feel renewed and reclaim your identity—or even a new one.

Next, change your wardrobe. Pack away the A-line tops and maternity pants (you just never know when you might need them again). You may not be back to "normal" yet, but you are getting there, so invest in a few pretty, front-opening tops that make you feel attractive and refreshed in your appearance.

Join a gym with a baby nursery, which will give you a couple of hours to focus on yourself. You need a little selfishness to stay sane. Don't lose sight of you.

BEAUTY RITUALS

Devise some new energizing beauty rituals.
□ Add a total of 6 drops of geranium, lavender, and vetiver together in a spray bottle of water. Use it as your wake-up spray whenever you feel tired and weary. It smells divine. Use it in place of your perfume to make you feel good.
□ Get your body back into condition with some luxurious treats. Use salt body scrubs and luscious body creams. Moisturize your breasts to keep them supple during the next few months of feeding.
□ Pamper your fingers and toes (see pages 56–57). You are in the house more for the first few weeks, so pad around barefoot and paint your toenails scarlet.

CALM AND CONTENTMENT

Practice meditation techniques to help you keep calm during this emotionally draining time. Choose a quiet half-hour while your baby is asleep. Close the curtains, sit comfortably without straining your back, rest your hands in your lap, close your eyes, and breath deeply.
□ Focus on your breathing, feeling the rise and fall of your abdomen with each breath. Silently count each breath in and out: one, in and out; two, in and out; and so on, up to ten. Then begin again and continue until everyday thoughts and anxieties no longer concern you.
□ Stop counting and repeat the pattern of breathing in and out, in and out, in and out. Let your mind dwell on the beauty of life. Your breath is the rhythm of life—the ebb and flow of the sea and the air and the days.
□ End with the kind of calm, peaceful, balanced breath that you would like to impart to your new baby. If you focus on the positive—the baby's future, your future together—you will bring new energy to the experience.
□ Practice this as often as you get the chance; it will become easier over time.

YOU AND YOUR BABY

This is a great time to start getting your body and mind back in balance, at the same time as giving your baby a good start in life.
□ Seek out a natural therapist. Reflexology, osteopathy, acupuncture, aromatherapy or homeopathy can all

help make you feel stronger and less emotional from within, using your body's own healing powers. That way, you and your baby both benefit safely.

□ Join a baby massage or baby yoga class. Massage can help soothe restless babies and help to get them into a good sleep pattern. It helps calm mothers down, too, giving you a bit of quiet time together. Baby yoga will teach you how to handle your baby with confidence and encourage your baby to feel comfortable with its own body. Classes also get you out of the house, meeting other women with babies of a similar age.

□ Keep a bottle of rosemary essential oil in your bag. Open it and inhale three times whenever you feel unable to focus on lots of different tasks at once.

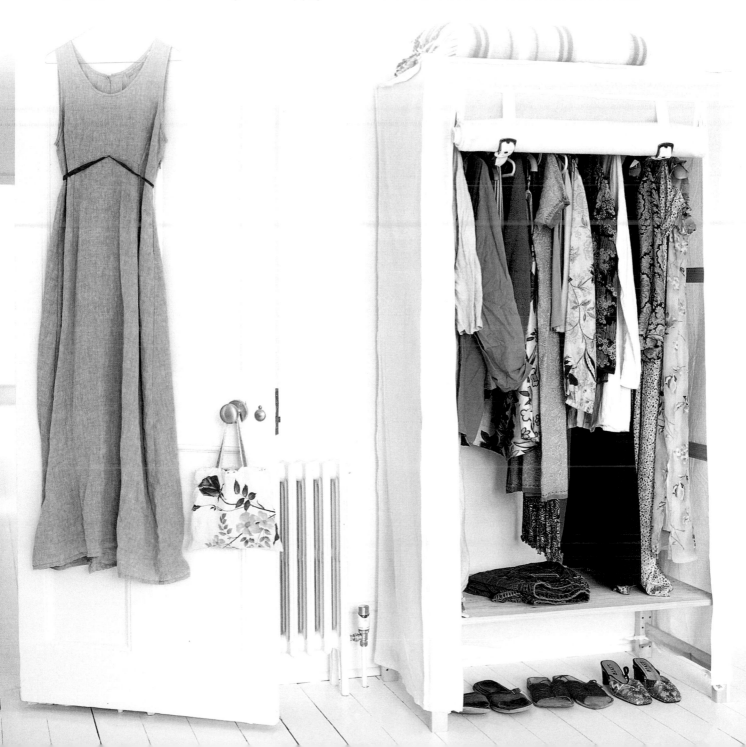

resources

Health of mother and baby
American Academy of
    Pediatrics
141 Northwest Point Blvd
Elk Grove Village
IL 60007-1098
847-434-4000
www.aap.org

KidsHealth.org
A good all-round website
for parents, reviewed by
doctors and sponsored by
The Nemours Foundation
Center for Children's Health.

Maternity Center Association
281 Park Avenue South
5th Floor
New York
NY 10010
212-777-5000
www.maternitywise.org
Aims to promote safe,
effective, and satisfying
maternity care for all
women and their children.

Midwife/doula referrals
Association of Labor Assistants
    and Childbirth Educators
P.O. Box 382724
Cambridge
MA 02074
617-441-2500
www.alace.org

The Bradley Method of
    Natural Childbirth
Box 5224
Sherman Oaks
CA 91413-5224
800-4-A-BIRTH
www.bradleybirth.com

Childbirth and Postpartum
    Professional Association
P.O. Box 491448
Lawrenceville
GA 30049
1-888-MY-CAPPA
www.cappa.net

Doulas of North America
P.O. Box 626
Jasper
IN 47547
801-756-7331
www.dona.org.

Doula World:
www.doulaworld.com.

International Childbirth
    Education Association
P.O. Box 20048
Minneapolis
MN 55420
952-854-8660
www.icea.org

Midwives Alliance of
    North America
4805 Lawrenceville Hwy
Suite 116-279
Lilburn
GA 30047
888-923-6262
www.mana.org

Breastfeeding support
Academy of Breast-feeding
    Medicine
191 Clarksville Road
Princeton Junction
NJ 08550
877-836-9947
www.bfmed.org

Baby Milk Action
www.babymilkaction.org

La Leche League
P.O. Box 4079
Schaumburg
IL 60168-4079
847-519-7730
www.lalecheleague.org

www.breastfeeding.com
A good all-purpose
breastfeeding support site.

Safety information
U.S. Health and Human
    Services
www.dshs.wa.gov/geninfo/
babysafe.html

Food and Drug Administration
5600 Fishers Lane
Rockville
MD 20857
888-463-6332
www.fda.gov

National Center on Birth
    Defects and Developmental
    Disabilities
www.cdc.gov/ncbdd
Works to promote health
in pregnancy and prevent birth
defects.

architects and designers whose work appears in this book

Marino + Giolito
Architecture/Interior Design
161 West 16th Street
New York, NY 10011
212-675-5737
marino.giolito@rcn.com
Page 92l.

Bruno Tanquerel
Artist
2 Passage St Sébastien
75011 Paris
France
+33 1 43 57 03 93
Page 111.

"Of all nature's gifts to the
human race, what is sweeter
to a man than his children?"

MARCUS TULLIUS CICERO

index

Numbers in **bold** indicate main references.

acne 19
active birth 120
acupressure 21, 35
acupuncture 99, 106, 111
alcohol 28–29, 32
allergies 32, 65
amino acids 50
antacids 98
antioxidants 66
anxiety 42–43, 60, **106**
arnica cream 129
aromatherapy 20, **60–61**
  for anxiety 43, 106
  for breastfeeding 132–33
  calming 45
  for constipation 99
  for depression 135
  energizing 22
  facial blends 55, 95
  facial massage 90–91
  for faintness 101
  foot soak 57
  hand soak 79
  for insomnia 106
  for itchy skin 82
  for labor 111, 122, 123
  for pampering 23
  for positivity 79
  postnatal 135, 138, 139
  relaxing 45, 108
  for scarring 53
  seductive 75
  to induce sleep 97
  for healing stitches 129
asthma 29
atomizer 55
avocado 66
Ayurveda 123

baby blues 135
Bach Flower Remedies 42, 43, 106, 122
back problems 36, 39
Balance Blend (essential oils) 61
banana 66
bath blends (essential oils)
  for anxiety 106
  bathing with baby 129
  for itchy skin 52
  for labor 119
  for pampering 23
  relaxing 106, 109

seductive 75
bathing 106
beanbags 71, 90, 97
birth
  planning 110, 121
  see also labor
bladder infections 101
bleeding 27, 63
  and sex 74
  and smoking 29
blood pressure
  high 40
  low 101
blood tests 27
body temperature 55, 63, 93, 94
  and bathing 106
  and exercise 40
bowel movements (postnatal) 136
brain development 31, 45
bras 14, 17, 93
Braxton-Hicks contractions 101
breastfeeding 129, **130–33**, 135
  at birth 121, 127
  and exercise 136
  and hair care 51
  and skin care 93
  the sugar trap 32
  and water 29
breasts 14, 41, 93
  sore nipples 129
breathing 45, 78
  in labor 121
  relaxation exercises 79, 90, 97, 108, 138
breech births 127
brushing the skin 22

calcium 86
calendula ointment 129
carrier oils 61
cellulite 22, 87
cervix, dilation of 111, 118
  encouraging 122
cesarean section 121, 127, 136
chamomile
  ointment 129, 132
  tea 106
chlorine 41
chorionic villus sampling (CVS) 10, 27, 63
clothes
  for coolness 94
  hiding the bump 25
  in the third trimester 82
coffee 28
colic 129

colostrum 82, 130
coloring hair 51
color therapy
  for positivity (orange) 79
  Reiki exercise 23
  for relaxation (blue) 108
communicating with your baby 78, 79
conception 10
constipation (postnatal) 136
contact lenses 88
contractions 118, **119**
  aromatherapy/herbalism for 122
  Braxton-Hicks 101
  and breathing 121
  positions for comfort 124
cooling down 94–5
cramp 86
cystic fibrosis 63
cystitis 101

dehydration (in baby) 133
dental work 92
diabetes 31, 32, 102
diaper rash 93
diet **30–33**
  and breastfeeding 133
  and cellulite 87
  and constipation 99
  and dental problems 92
  energy foods **64–66**
  and healthy hair 50
  and mood swings 135
  and morning sickness 35
dietary supplements 10, 31, 64, 66, 86
digestion
  heartburn 98
  improving 65
docosohexaenoic acid (DHA) 31
dry body brushing 22

edema see swelling
estrogen 18, 19, 43, 50
Elemis 71
emotions 14, 42–43
  postnatal 135
energy diet 64–66
engorgement 130–32
epidurals 119, 127
episiotomies 127
  healing 129
exercise **39–41**
  to prepare for labor **104–105**
  to minimize leg swelling 85

postnatal 136
  to reduce stress 43
  yoga **71–73**
eyeglasses 88
eyes 25, 55, **88–89**
  exercising 109
  eye masks 23

face massage 90
facial spray 95
fainting 101
fake tan 82
fathers see partners
feet 57, 87, 94, 95
  massage 109
fennel tea 133
fetal alcohol syndrome 28
Filderman, Janet 25
fish oil 31
fluid retention (swelling) 39, 40, 85, 88
folic acid 10, 66
food
  allergies 32
  what to avoid 32, 35
  see also diet
foot care 57
forceps 127
fruit smoothies 66

Gabriel, Noella 20, 60, 71
genetic disorders 63
ginger 35
gum problems 92

hair **50–51**
  scalp massage 77, 79
hand care 56–57
heartburn 98
hemorrhoids 99
herbal tinctures 122
hiding the bump 25
high blood pressure 40
homeopathic remedies
  for anxiety 106
  for bruising 129
  for constipation 99
  for cramp 86
  for gum problems 92
  for labor 123
  for poor milk flow 133
  for morning sickness 35
  for pain 111
Hypercal 92, 129

incontinence, stress 68, 101
insomnia 60, **106**

author's acknowledgments

Thank you first of all, to my lovely husband, Jim, without whom I would never have had the experience to write this book; and to my three very dear children, Olivia, William, and Phoebe—for whom I hope this book will be a testament to how much I love, and have loved, having you. Thank you to Fiona Lindsay of Limelight Management, my wonderful agent, and to Alison Starling at Ryland Peters & Small for wanting this book almost as much as I. A special thank you also to the editor, Henrietta Heald, and the designer, Sally Powell, at Ryland Peters & Small for their endless patience. To aromatherapists Noella Gabriel of Elemis and Glenda Taylor for sharing their expertise; trichologist Glen Lyons of Philip Kingsley Trichological Centre in London; and especially to Leslie Spires, Senior Midwife at The Active Birth Centre, Queen Charlotte's & Chelsea Hospital, London, who greatly reinforced my belief that a happy positive woman has a happier, more positive birth. And lastly to my friends and mothers: Nancy Brady, Diana Collier, Catherine Everest, Kate Harris, Sheena Miller, Ingrid Ryder, and Suzanne Wilson, who have kindly shared many of their experiences to help me create this book.

publisher's acknowledgments

The publishers would like to say thanks to all our models, especially Sarah and Max, as well as Jodie, baby Dylan, and Nikki. Thanks also to Neal's Yard Remedies and to Noella Gabriel, Director of Product and Treatment Development at Elemis.

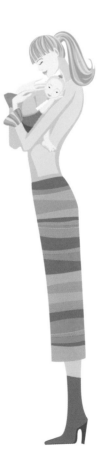

photography credits

Jacket photography: front jacket and back jacket above by DEBI TRELOAR; back jacket below by DAN DUCHARS.

Photography by DAN DUCHARS unless otherwise stated.
Key: a=above, b=below, r=right, l=left, c=center.

MARTIN BRIGDALE 66l; DAVID BRITTAIN 23b; PETER CASSIDY 32c, 33, 65r; CHRIS EVERARD 92l New York City apartment designed by Marino + Giolito, 111 an apartment in Paris designed by Bruno Tanquerel; WILLIAM LINGWOOD 30r, 34, 50b, 64a, 67, 95a; DAVID MONTGOMERY 3, 5 background, 14, 18l, 20, 21, 22, 23a, 25, 26, 27, 29, 45b, 52, 54, 55b, 56r, 57, 60, 74 background, 76 background, 78, 79, 86, 87, 92r, 93, 94b, 107, 122, 123, 133r; DEBI TRELOAR 1, 4, 5, 16, 17, 19r, 24, 28, 30l, 32l & r, 38, 41, 43, 44b, 45a, 50a, 53, 56l & c, 58, 59, 62, 64b, 65l & c, 66 c & r, 69, 70, 71, 74 inset, 76 inset, 77l, 83, 84, 88, 94a, 95b, 98 inset, 104, 105, 110, 112, 113, 115, 119, 126, 127, 128, 133l, 134 background, 139, 140, 141; POLLY WREFORD 8, 11, 12, 42l, 47, 77r, 85, 137; FRANCESCA YORKE 31, 92 background, 98 background.